Regulating Medicines in a Globalized World

THE NEED FOR INCREASED RELIANCE AMONG REGULATORS

Alastair J. Wood and Patricia Cuff, *Editors*

Committee on Mutual Recognition Agreements and Reliance in the Regulation of Medicines

Board on Global Health

Health and Medicine Division

A Consensus Study Report of

The National Academies of
SCIENCES · ENGINEERING · MEDICINE

THE NATIONAL ACADEMIES PRESS
Washington, DC
www.nap.edu

THE NATIONAL ACADEMIES PRESS **500 Fifth Street, NW** **Washington, DC 20001**

This activity was supported by a contract between the National Academy of Sciences and the U.S. Food and Drug Administration's Office of International Programs (HHSP233201400020B). Any opinions, findings, conclusions, or recommendations expressed in this publication do not necessarily reflect the views of any organization or agency that provided support for the project.

International Standard Book Number-13: 978-0-309-49863-0
International Standard Book Number-10: 0-309-49863-5
Digital Object Identifier: https://doi.org/10.17226/25594
Library of Congress Control Number: 2020930367

Additional copies of this publication are available from the National Academies Press, 500 Fifth Street, NW, Keck 360, Washington, DC 20001; (800) 624-6242 or (202) 334-3313; http://www.nap.edu.

Printed in the United States of America

Suggested citation: National Academies of Sciences, Engineering, and Medicine. 2020. *Regulating medicines in a globalized world: The need for increased reliance among regulators*. Washington, DC: The National Academies Press. https://doi.org/10.17226/25594.

The National Academies of
SCIENCES · ENGINEERING · MEDICINE

The **National Academy of Sciences** was established in 1863 by an Act of Congress, signed by President Lincoln, as a private, nongovernmental institution to advise the nation on issues related to science and technology. Members are elected by their peers for outstanding contributions to research. Dr. Marcia McNutt is president.

The **National Academy of Engineering** was established in 1964 under the charter of the National Academy of Sciences to bring the practices of engineering to advising the nation. Members are elected by their peers for extraordinary contributions to engineering. Dr. John L. Anderson is president.

The **National Academy of Medicine** (formerly the Institute of Medicine) was established in 1970 under the charter of the National Academy of Sciences to advise the nation on medical and health issues. Members are elected by their peers for distinguished contributions to medicine and health. Dr. Victor J. Dzau is president.

The three Academies work together as the **National Academies of Sciences, Engineering, and Medicine** to provide independent, objective analysis and advice to the nation and conduct other activities to solve complex problems and inform public policy decisions. The National Academies also encourage education and research, recognize outstanding contributions to knowledge, and increase public understanding in matters of science, engineering, and medicine.

Learn more about the National Academies of Sciences, Engineering, and Medicine at **www.nationalacademies.org.**

The National Academies of
SCIENCES · ENGINEERING · MEDICINE

COMMITTEE ON MUTUAL RECOGNITION AGREEMENTS AND RELIANCE IN THE REGULATION OF MEDICINES

ALASTAIR J. J. WOOD (*Chair*), Professor of Medicine (*Emeritus*), Professor of Pharmacology (*Emeritus*), Vanderbilt University
DAVID W. BEIER, Managing Director, Bay City Capital
THOMAS J. BOLLYKY, Director, Global Health Program, Council on Foreign Relations
KATHERINE C. BOND, Vice President, International Public Policy and Regulatory Affairs, U.S. Pharmacopeia
MARTHA A. BRUMFIELD, President and Chief Executive Officer (*Former*), Critical Path Institute
DAVID COCKBURN, Head of Manufacturing and Quality Compliance (*Retired*), European Medicines Agency
ELIZABETH GOLBERG, Senior Fellow (*Former*), Mossavar-Rahmani Center for Business and Government, Harvard Kennedy School
LAWRENCE O. GOSTIN, Linda D. & Timothy J. O'Neill Professor of Global Health Law, Georgetown University
GAVIN HUNTLEY-FENNER, Human Factors and Safety Consultant, Huntley-Fenner Advisors, Inc.
BARBARA KOREMENOS, Professor, University of Michigan
MURRAY LUMPKIN, Deputy Director, Global Health/Integrated Development, Lead for Global Regulatory Systems Initiatives, Bill & Melinda Gates Foundation
LEMBIT RÄGO, Secretary-General, Council for International Organizations of Medical Sciences

Study Staff

PATRICIA CUFF, Study Director (*from April 2019*), Senior Program Officer
MONICA WHITLEY, Study Director (*until August 2019*)
DANIEL FLYNN, Research Associate
INEZ ADAMS, Research Assistant
KELLY CHOI, Senior Program Assistant (*from April 2019*)
NATALIE LUBIN, Senior Program Assistant (*until April 2019*)
JULIE PAVLIN, Director, Board on Global Health

Consultant

RONA BRIERE, Editor

Reviewers

This Consensus Study Report was reviewed in draft form by individuals chosen for their diverse perspectives and technical expertise. The purpose of this independent review is to provide candid and critical comments that will assist the National Academies of Sciences, Engineering, and Medicine in making each published report as sound as possible and to ensure that it meets the institutional standards for quality, objectivity, evidence, and responsiveness to the study charge. The review comments and draft manuscript remain confidential to protect the integrity of the deliberative process.

The committee thanks the following individuals for their review of this report:

ROBERT CALIFF, Duke University
EMER COOKE, World Health Organization
PETRA DOERR, Petra Doerr Consulting Ltd.
MARTIN HARVEY-ALLCHURCH, Unitaid Geneva
PAUL HUCKLE, GlaxoSmithKline (*Retired*)
IAN HUDSON, Medicines & Healthcare products Regulatory Agency
RAJ LONG, Bill & Melinda Gates Foundation
TOSHIYOSHI TOMINAGA, Japan Self-Medication Industry

Although the reviewers listed above provided many constructive comments and suggestions, they were not asked to endorse the conclusions or recommendations of this report nor did they see the final draft before its release. The review of this report was overseen by **JOSHUA M. SHARFSTEIN,** Johns Hopkins Bloomberg School of Public Health, and

WILLIAM M. SAGE, The University of Texas at Austin. They were responsible for making certain that an independent examination of this report was carried out in accordance with the standards of the National Academies and that all review comments were carefully considered. Responsibility for the final content rests entirely with the authoring committee and the National Academies.

Acknowledgments

During the course of this year-long study, the committee invited key participants from different countries to share their insights at open committee meetings and information-gathering sessions. This report would not have been possible without their important contributions. The committee would like to take this opportunity to thank all of those who gave generously of their time, knowledge, experience, and resources (see Appendix D). In particular, the committee would like to thank the Bill & Melinda Gates Foundation, which supported the committee's information-gathering session in London, and the U.S. Food and Drug Administration for sponsoring this study, with special thanks to Mark Abdoo, Russell Campbell, and Mary Lou Valdez. The committee would be remiss if it did not acknowledge the contributions of the National Academies staff, including administrative assistance from Kelly Choi and Natalie Lubin, research help from Inez Adams and Daniel Flynn, oversight from Julie Pavlin and Monica Whitley, and overall study coordination and direction from Patricia Cuff. Similar appreciation goes to the talented editing staff headed by Rona Briere and supported by Alisa Decatur. It is through the participation of all of these valued stakeholders that the committee presents this study report stemming from the input and efforts of everyone involved.

Preface

Globalization is now an integral part of all of our lives. We routinely expect to be able to perform many aspects of our everyday activities regardless of where we are. We step off an international flight in some far-flung destination and expect to instantly use our cell phone, order a ride hailing service, pay for a hotel with our credit card, access our electronic documents held on a distant server, and even withdraw cash from our local bank account while traveling to faraway lands. Just as our lives have been touched by the power of globalization, so, too, has the pharmaceutical industry. Drug development, authorization, and regulatory supervision have become international endeavors, with most medicines now being global commodities.

Drug companies operate in many parts of the world, utilize global supply chains that often include facilities in countries with weaker regulations than those of the United States, perform pivotal trials in multiple countries to support registration submissions in multiple jurisdictions, and subsequently market their medicines throughout most of the world. However, they are then regulated by individual national regulators, each of which requires submissions for review prior to marketing authorization. Each review procedure requires resources on the part of the sponsor and of the regulatory authorities, and often there is little acknowledgment that a similar product review is occurring, sometimes simultaneously, in several other countries. All of these national regulators have the mission of ensuring that drugs authorized for use in their countries are safe, effective, and appropriate for their health care system and their population. The standards for such safety, efficacy, and quality judgments among the major well-resourced regulators (the U.S. Food and Drug Administration [FDA]; the European Medicines Agency; the Pharmaceuticals and Medical Devices Agency, Japan; Health Canada; the Medicines & Healthcare products Regulatory Agency, UK; Swissmedic; and the Therapeutic Goods Administration, Australia) are well known and similar, if not identical. Although the final judgment on whether to approve a drug for marketing is an important sovereign decision for each national regulator to make, based on what is appropriate and what level of risk tolerance exists in a given society, in some cases much of the work that forms the scientific basis for the authorization decision is quite similar, if not identical, across the various regulators. The result is considerable duplicative and redundant work being performed throughout the world, which benefits neither national nor global public health. For example, having multiple regulators inspecting the same manufacturing site has little value and in fact may compromise public health because the time might better be devoted to inspecting different sites and therefore ensuring the safety of a larger spectrum of manufacturing sites. Clearly if different versions of a product are manufactured by the same company at different sites for different markets, inspections of the different sites are required. Similarly, multiple detailed reviews of exactly the same data by multiple national reviewers are unlikely to improve knowledge of the product or patient outcomes. In this context, the purpose of this FDA-requested study was for an expert committee convened by the National Academies of Sciences, Engineering, and Medicine to consider the role of mutual recognition and other reliance activities among regulators in contributing to enhancing public health.

Through its conversations with various key stakeholders, the committee came to recognize that two very different roles exist for national regulators in relation to reliance activities. First, there is the potential for horizontal reliance activities. These are activities conducted among well-resourced regulators who share similar regulatory and scientific skillsets, as well as regulatory and structural similarities, that can more easily give way to mutual confidence and bidirectional reliance. It was within such reliance activities that committee members saw opportunities for more effective public health protection by improving and expanding the potential for relying on the work of other similar regulatory authorities for making informed decisions.

Additional opportunities for leveraging reliance activities more broadly have the potential to impact public health globally. This was the concept envisioned by members of the committee, who proposed greater access by less-resourced regulators to the regulatory work products (e.g., inspection reports, scientific assessments) of well-resourced regulators. In this way, less-resourced regulators would be better positioned to make informed sovereign regulatory decisions, while using their own finite resources in the most efficient manner. Reliance in these scenarios might be unidirectional, but at present such reliance often is not possible because of the unwillingness or inability of some national regulators to share unredacted or less-redacted work products. Lack of access to such work products has direct negative impacts on the global health of millions of patients, especially those outside of Europe, North America, and Oceania.

The committee also recognized that as medicines, such as biologicals and biosimilars, become increasingly more complex and as cell-based and genetic therapies become more widespread, only a limited number of national regulators will be able to deploy the full range of skills necessary for comprehensive reviews of such products. Thus, it becomes imperative that reviews of complex medicines be made available to other regulators so they can provide appropriate oversight of these products in their jurisdictions. Addressing these challenges is a high priority for global health, one that requires the attention of both national regulators and legislators to facilitate the ability of others to use the work products of well-resourced regulators.

The committee considered the opportunities that increased reliance activities by regulatory authorities might provide for the national and global public health, but also considered the practical difficulties of implementing such activities. Global regulators have been working diligently in the International Council for Harmonisation of Technical Requirements for Pharmaceuticals for Human Use and other fora to develop and agree on harmonized technical standards for the registration of medicines. As with so many of the things we now take for granted that function seamlessly across national frontiers, there are opportunities for improvements in medicines regulation that could enhance global health. However, it is worth emphasizing that the committee did not see this exercise as necessarily being one that would reduce costs, but rather one that could enhance public health by allowing the most efficient deployment of scarce and precious global regulatory resources.

Contents

Boxes, Figures, and Table

BOXES

FIGURES

TABLE

Acronyms and Abbreviations

ACSS	Australia-Canada-Singapore-Switzerland Consortium
API	active pharmaceutical ingredient
ASEAN	Association of Southeast Asian Nations
CBER	Center for Biologics Evaluation and Research
CC	confidentiality commitment
CFR	Code of Federal Regulations
COFEPRIS	Comisión Federal para la Protección contra Riesgos Sanitarious (Federal Commission for the Protection against Sanitary Risks) (Mexico)
CRS	Caribbean Regulatory System
EEA	European Economic Area
EMA	European Medicines Agency
EU	European Union
FDA	U.S. Food and Drug Administration
GAO	Government Accountability Office
GCP	good clinical practice
GLP	good laboratory practice
GMP	good manufacturing practice
GPvP	good pharmacovigilance practice
ICDRA	International Conference of Drug Regulatory Authorities

ICH	International Council for Harmonisation of Technical Requirements for Pharmaceuticals for Human Use
ICMRA	International Coalition of Medicines Regulatory Authorities
IPRP	International Pharmaceutical Regulators Programme
MOC	Memorandum of Cooperation
MOU	Memorandum of Understanding
MRA	mutual recognition agreement
NHP	natural health product
OECD	Organisation for Economic Co-operation and Development
PBRER	periodic benefit/risk evaluation report
PIC/S	Pharmaceutical Inspection Co-operation Scheme
PSUR	periodic safety update report
PV	pharmacovigilance
RA	regulatory authority
TGA	Therapeutic Goods Administration (Australia)
UK	United Kingdom
VICH	International Cooperation on Harmonisation of Technical Requirements for Registration of Veterinary Medicinal Products
WHO	World Health Organization

Summary

Patients and health care providers expect quality-assured, safe, and effective medicines that are properly labeled for the purposes for which they have been approved. A key objective of medicines regulatory authorities is to promote and protect public health by ensuring the quality, safety, and efficacy of medicines and by ensuring that they are properly labeled based on robust science. Fulfilling this mission in a time of rapid scientific change, increasing complexity of medicines, and globalization of production and product supply chains has presented regulatory authorities with multiple challenges while also opening doors to opportunities in the form of greater regulatory cooperation and information sharing among the regulators.

It was in this context that the U.S. Food and Drug Administration's (FDA's) Office of International Programs (now the Office of Global Policy and Strategy) asked the National Academies of Sciences, Engineering, and Medicine to convene an ad hoc committee of experts to conduct a landscape review of the tools (e.g., recognition and other regulatory arrangements) being used by regulators to help them oversee the quality, safety, and efficacy of medicines throughout the product lifecycle (from initial development through marketing approval and distribution). Along with this landscape, the committee's Statement of Task outlined requests to analyze interagency recognition and other forms of reliance in terms of major challenges and opportunities as well as potential risks and benefits. To carry out its charge, the committee held a series of information-gathering sessions along with two open meetings at which the committee heard from representatives of industry, patient groups, international organizations, and regulatory authorities. These informants' comments were supplemented by written feedback from a targeted group of regulators; a comprehensive literature search; and online information, mainly in the form of government-issued reports. With this collective input, as well as recognition of the common public health mission of all regulatory authorities, the committee synthesized two key messages. These key messages serve as the lens through which the committee's conclusion and recommendations should be viewed:

- Regulation through recognition and reliance arrangements is now a 21st-century best regulatory practice. Accordingly, regulators, regardless of human, technical, and financial resources, need to make increased use of reliance and cooperation with other trusted regulators, as no regulator has the resources it needs to meet all of its public health responsibilities.
- Impediments to regulators entering into and using such informal and formal recognition and reliance arrangements to help them obtain the information they need for their regulatory decision making should be removed.

In addition to and based on its one conclusion, the committee formulated six recommendations, the first of which includes a strategy for improving regulatory cooperation[1] that places the public's health at the center of collaboration efforts. The strategy targets multiple stakeholder groups with an expressed interest in public health and patient care. Within this strategy, each group is called on to play a role in enhancing regulatory cooperation in the form of recognition and reliance arrangements that range from informal, collaborative activities to the most formal—a mutual recognition agreement (MRA). It is safe to say that virtually all regulatory authorities are motivated by a public health mission to safeguard their populations with respect to the medicines coming into, and currently on, the market in their jurisdictions. Additionally, given the rapid movement of people and illnesses across borders in today's world, it is similarly safe to say that public health is a global concern and that all regulators, regardless of size or financial resources, exercise their responsibilities within that global public health framework as part of a larger global regulatory enterprise. How regulatory authorities carry out their missions and structure their regulatory cooperation activities is often a function of human and financial resources. In this report, and as reflected in the recommended strategy, regulatory authorities are divided into three categories: well-resourced, moderately well-resourced, and lower-resourced.

[1]Regulatory cooperation is considered by the committee to be any formal or informal interaction with another regulator for the purposes of sharing information or working together toward a common goal.

ROLE OF REGULATORY AUTHORITIES

The core functions of regulatory authorities include ensuring that products released for use in their jurisdiction are properly evaluated and meet appropriate standards of quality, safety, and efficacy that are maintained throughout all stages of the product lifecycle and supply chain, including manufacturing, production, packaging, and distribution (WHO, 2019g). These basic functions must be met while enabling timely access to quality-assured products and encouraging innovation (WHO, 2019e). It is industry's responsibility to comply with rules and scientific and technical standards established for products, and it is the regulator's responsibility to oversee compliance with these rules and standards (Rönninger et al., 2012) and to work with the larger community to develop new standards as technology and scientific knowledge improve. For medicines (the focus of this report), there are regulations describing compliance activities and good practices across the medicines lifecycle from preclinical research to post-marketing surveillance. Guidance is provided by regulatory authorities at each stage (as shown in Figure S-1), but it is up to industry to interpret the guidance and apply it to their situations. Good laboratory practice (GLP) sets guidelines for ensuring that laboratory data are of high quality and reliable in the preclinical phase; good clinical practice (GCP) guides aspects of studies involving human subjects; good manufacturing practice (GMP) provides guidance for the manufacturing, production, and distribution of medicines; and good pharmacovigilance practice (GPvP) provides guidance for the appropriate oversight of products once they have been released onto the general market. Assuring an overall positive benefit/risk profile to the most appropriate level possible is essential throughout the entire medicine product lifecycle.

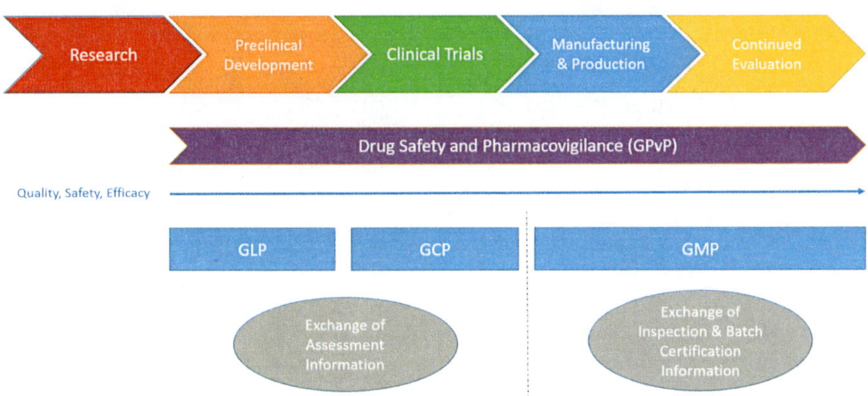

FIGURE S-1 Lifecycle of a medicine.

For the purposes of this report, regulatory work products are the administrative documents produced by a regulator as a result of a regulatory authority's evaluation. These work products might include an inspection report or certificate of compliance for GMP, official batch release, or an assessment report regarding evaluation of the clinical and statistical elements of the clinical data used in the application requesting approval to market a new medicine.

Sponsors of new drugs create a registration dossier (e.g., "marketing authorization application," "new drug application") that is submitted to a regulatory authority for assessment regarding possible approval for marketing. It will typically include information from the sponsor's product development program, such as data purporting to demonstrate the overall positive benefit/risk profile of the product, including its safety and effectiveness in clinical studies; the preclinical laboratory data; and the data surrounding the manufacture of the product. If the product is approved for marketing, regulatory authorities will continue to oversee its manufacture and production and ongoing benefit/risk profile, often taking a risk-based approach to determine the level of intensity of that oversight. Each stage of the product lifecycle presents opportunities for the use of recognition and reliance between and among regulatory authorities. Often, the design and extent of such recognition and reliance are based on the availability of the regulatory authorities' technical resources.

RECOGNITION AND RELIANCE

As defined by the World Health Organization (WHO), recognition occurs when a regulatory authority accepts the regulatory decision of another authority "as its own decision." Reliance takes place when a regulatory authority takes into account the work products of another authority (e.g., inspection reports, scientific assessment reports, joint assessment reports produced together with another authority) to help inform the receiving authority's own regulatory decision, which in the end may differ from the decision made by the initial authority using the same work products. In essence, one could argue that recognition is a subset of reliance, or the "ultimate reliance." The important point is that even when an authority uses recognition or reliance, it has sovereignty over and responsibility for the regulatory decision it makes for its country—it does not "outsource" its decision making. A regulatory authority's decision to *routinely accept the regulatory decision of another authority* or to *take into account* the work products of another regulator to inform its decision making is the choice and responsibility of that regulatory authority. The decision to do so might be based on a variety of factors, including the context in which a regulatory decision is being made, access to technical or financial resources, and whether there is sufficient trust and confidence in the decision and/or work product/information of the regulatory authority being relied on.

Different tools to facilitate recognition and reliance across the product lifecycle are available. These are collectively referred to in this report as "arrangements." Arrangements can be more formal, established and implemented, for example, through Memoranda of Understanding, confidentiality commitments, and MRAs; or they can be informal arrangements through the establishment of ad hoc committees, working parties, and other, more topic-specific working groups (EMA, 2019g). WHO's draft guidelines for good regulatory practices note that "less formal practices include sharing of information, scientific collaboration, common risk assessments, joint reviews, and development of standards" (WHO, 2016b, p. 27).

Much attention has historically been focused on the use of recognition and reliance arrangements with respect to GMP inspections, while there has been less of a focus on GLP, GCP, and GPvP inspections or other aspects of regulatory decision making. These other areas may represent opportunities for future expansion of arrangements.

UNDERSTANDING THE REGULATORY ENVIRONMENT

In an environment of limited human and financial resources and at a time of unprecedented globalization and societal requests for faster approvals of drugs, medicines regulators have felt pressure to stretch their finite resources. To that end, they have undertaken a wide range of activities geared toward helping each other manage a growing workload by leveraging those limited resources. While a few regulatory authorities have access to higher levels of technical and financial resources, the vast majority of medicines regulatory authorities globally would be considered moderately well- to lower-resourced. In fact, WHO estimates that, based on the criteria in its Global Benchmarking Tool, approximately 100 of the 194 WHO member states do not have a medicines regulatory agency that is technically capacitated to meet even the basic requirements of a medicines regulatory authority (Khadem, 2019). For many regulatory authorities, relying on the work of other trusted regulators is the only way to keep pace with the growing demand for their services. This was the overwhelming message of regulators in Australia, Canada, Singapore, and Switzerland who have joined together through a work-sharing project based on trust and confidence built among the partners. Pilot tests, working groups, and other convening activities designed to build trust and confidence are often essential first steps toward relying on the work of other regulators. If trust and confidence are satisfactorily built, authorities may consider engaging in formal and/or informal recognition or reliance arrangements, the most formal of which are MRAs. Figure S-2 shows how trust and confidence are

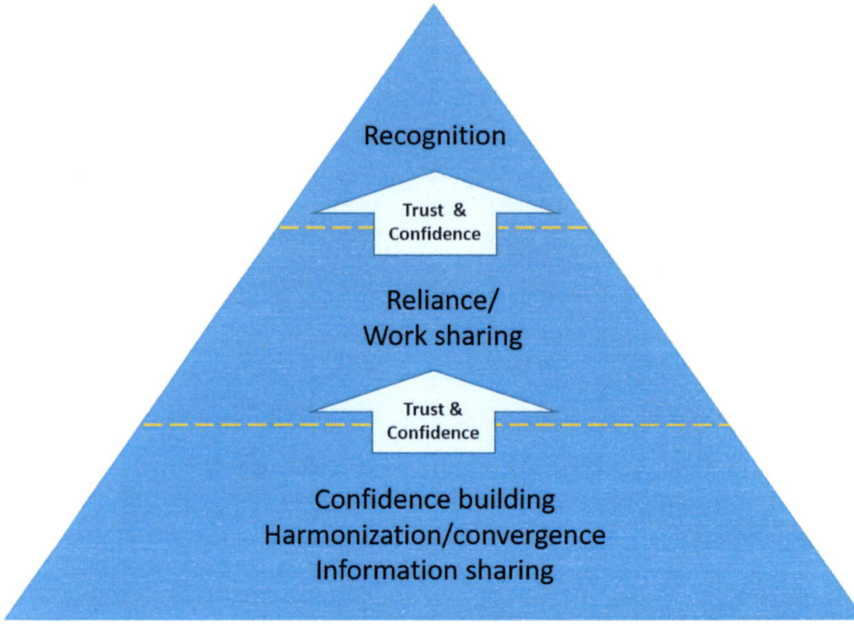

FIGURE S-2 Building confidence and trust from and for greater reliance.
SOURCES: Adapted from a figure created by Dr. Petra Doerr, Swissmedic, and presented by Emer Cooke, World Health Organization (WHO, 2019i).

necessary for all forms of recognition and reliance arrangements (mutual and others).

There are currently 14 MRAs for medicines, listed in Appendix B of this report. While less formal reliance arrangements promote the sharing of information and facilitate fewer redundant inspections and other regulatory activities, MRAs allow regulatory authorities not just to rely on each other's work products but to recognize them officially as equivalent to their own. However, this is possible only if shared reports are complete and essentially free from redactions. Current medicines regulatory MRAs are limited primarily to GMP reports and official batch release reports, although a few also include GLP reports. To progress beyond GMP and expand the classes of products subject to the GMP MRAs, regulators would likely have to establish high levels of trust and confidence by building a track record of demonstrated equivalence. In the meantime, regulators use or could use other, more agile reliance tools to work with other regulators in managing their growing workloads to help ensure the quality, safety, efficacy, and availability of medicines.

LEVERAGING KEY OPPORTUNITIES TO OVERCOME MEDICINES REGULATORY CHALLENGES

Rapid globalization of drug discovery, development, manufacturing, and delivery has significant implications for public health. The resources required to assure comprehensive oversight of these activities is now an enormous task for even well-resourced national medicines regulatory authorities. All have limited resources to accomplish sufficiently all the tasks they are asked to perform. The ongoing evolution of the science and technologies associated with drug discovery, development, manufacturing, and delivery (e.g., dramatic increases in more complex biological medicines and emerging use of cell and gene therapies) poses additional capacity and expertise challenges for regulatory authorities. These challenges underscore the need for further cooperation and collaboration among authorities; however, achieving that cooperation can be difficult because individual authorities have different histories; legal frameworks; human, technical, and financial resources; and areas of expertise. In confronting the global challenges of medicines regulation, cooperation and collaboration among regulators offer opportunities to share information and increase the transparency of each other's activities; to share finite resources and address the growing workload resulting from globalization; and to rely on each other's processes, work products, and decision making via both formal reliance arrangements such as MRAs and other, less formal arrangements.

Based on its extensive deliberations and input from stakeholders representing regulatory authorities, international organizations, industry, and patient groups, the committee agreed that public health must be at the center of all medicines regulatory recognition and reliance arrangements. Additionally, regulatory authorities require the support of industry, patients, and governments to realize the maximum benefits of any recognition or reliance arrangement.

Conclusion: The committee concludes that protecting and promoting public health in a time of globalization and unprecedented advances in technology and medicines—which are mirrored by the growing complexity of medicines and the supply chains for their manufacture and production—is the single greatest challenge facing medicines regulatory authorities today. It is therefore imperative that regulatory authorities at all resource levels—well, moderately well, and lower—find ways to continue or expand on their ability and willingness to work together to maximize the use of their finite resources so they can ensure the quality, safety, efficacy, and availability of medicines for their jurisdictions in both emergency and non-emergency situations.

However, for regulatory authorities to build further on their current recognition and reliance activities, impediments to entering into and using formal and informal recognition and reliance arrangements need to be removed. Some impediments lie within the regulatory authority itself, while others may be external to the agency and influenced by those within policy, industry, or consumer/patient advocacy groups. Each of these stakeholder groups has a role to play in supporting efforts to enhance cooperation among regulatory authorities, with the overarching aim of improving public health. The committee therefore recommends that all regulatory authorities and other key stakeholder groups demonstrate their support for formal and informal medicines regulatory recognition and reliance arrangements using a targeted approach.

Recommendation 1: The committee recommends a strategy that leverages the support of each stakeholder group in the following manner:

- **All regulatory authorities, especially those that are well- and moderately well-resourced, should increase information sharing and the transparency of each other's regulatory activities across the lifecycle of medicines in ways that can facilitate more efficient resource allocation and decision making for all regulators and reduce the burden of redundant regulatory activities on regulators, patients, and industry.**
- **All regulatory authorities, especially those that are well- and moderately well-resourced, should be allowed to share their work products in essentially unredacted form (i.e., full reports without parts of the report expunged, except for personal privacy information) with other regulatory authorities so assessment and inspection information can be made available to those other regulators, especially those that are lower-resourced, thereby enabling access to quality, usable regulatory information by a greater number of regulatory authorities for addressing global public health needs. In this respect, policy makers, and the U.S. Congress in particular, should weigh the challenges and opportunities involved in empowering their respective medicines regulatory authorities to share complete, unredacted inspection reports (e.g., good manufacturing practice reports) with other regulatory authorities so as to facilitate learning, aid in decision making, reduce the use of limited resources on redundant inspections, decrease the burden on industry of redundant inspections, and strengthen the overall global public heath infrastructure for safe and effective quality medicines.**
- **Lower-resourced regulatory authorities should consider the risks and benefits of unilateral recognition of the regulatory decisions**

of trusted regulatory authorities when doing so would facilitate better public health decision making in the context in which the lower-resourced regulatory authority functions.

- **Industry should support the recognition and reliance efforts of regulatory authorities by encouraging them to share less redacted or, better, unredacted reports with their trusted regulatory authority partners, and by showing a willingness to share health-related data and/or information relevant to regulatory decision making more publicly to benefit the global public health good and reduce the sharing authority's own burden of redundant oversight.**
- **Patient and consumer groups should support the recognition and reliance efforts of medicines regulatory authorities by advocating for a "public health protection and promotion" framing of all such arrangements and for their increased use.**

The committee further believes, based on its information gathering and expert opinion, that formal and informal recognition and reliance arrangements are highly effective tools for facilitating cooperation and reliance on the work of other regulatory authorities, when they are established in ways that emphasize public health, maximize efficiencies, reduce the burden of redundancy, and have the potential to benefit both global and national public health by ensuring effective and efficient access to safe and effective quality medicines.

Improving Public Health Through Better Designed MRAs

MRAs are one tool to facilitate the regulatory cooperation that can enable regulators to better fulfill their regulatory public health mandates. MRAs developed through trade agreements—which can include a wide range of commodities such as electrical goods and telecom equipment—can be slow to conclude and costly for administrators, regulators, and negotiators in terms of time and human resources (Correia de Brito et al., 2016). If the primary objective of these agreements that involve medicines is to improve public health, it stands to reason that medicines regulators, with their shared understanding of public health, are key to developing and designing such agreements. MRAs have usually been developed in the context of trade negotiations, with the dual aim of reducing technical barriers to trade and promoting public health. To prioritize what should be the public health aims and focus of these arrangements, the committee believes that medicines regulators, with their public health background, are ideally positioned to increase the scope and substance of interagency reliance. Medicines regulators share a common interest, namely, improving the public's health through the availability of safe and effective medicines.

That shared, common interest makes medicines regulators well suited to developing, designing, and implementing the substance of such regulatory agreements in the future. Therefore, the committee makes the following recommendation.

Recommendation 2: Policy makers, including lawmakers, should explore empowering regulators to expand the scope and substance of future mutual recognition agreements (MRAs) that address issues related to the safety, efficacy, and manufacturing quality of medicines, and to ensure that these MRAs are designed, developed, and implemented primarily by medicines regulators. Policy makers will also need to ensure that regulators have adequate resources for these tasks.[2]

Responding to Evolving Science and Technology

MRAs, as currently designed, are not sufficiently agile tools to respond to the rapid pace at which science, technology, and the global medicines regulatory enterprise are all evolving. More agile reliance arrangements would be better suited to meet these challenges. To address the challenges associated with the globalized production of medicines, as well as the growing need to address the medicine requirements during public health emergencies, the committee believes that MRAs and other reliance arrangements should be expanded to include new areas.

Recommendation 3: The committee recommends that regulators consider increasing the current scope of both formal and less formal reliance arrangements, including mutual recognition agreements, and that policy makers encourage regulatory authorities to explore formal and informal opportunities for reliance arrangements with other trusted regulatory authorities that give regulators greater flexibility in responding to challenges that affect their responsibility in overseeing the quality, safety, and efficacy of medicines throughout the medicines' lifecycle. Potential areas identified for such expansion of scope include good laboratory practice, good clinical practice, and good pharmacovigilance practice inspection reports; preclinical assessment reports;

[2]Murray Lumpkin, Lembit Rago, and Katherine Bond did not fully concur with this recommendation because they believe it still leaves the negotiation, oversight, and finalization of MRAs related to medicines regulation to trade negotiators, rather than empowering medicines regulators to design, develop, conclude, and implement these specific medicines regulatory MRAs on their own. They believe that is the only way to ensure that public health is the sole focus of the negotiation and agreement and that the agreement is negotiated and concluded in the collaborative public health atmosphere that exists among medicines regulators and not the competitive business dynamic that pervades and shades trade negotiations.

bioequivalence assessment reports; and a wider scope of product classes covered by such arrangements.

Better Utilization of the European Union (EU)-US Mutual Recognition Agreement

The EU-US MRA, as currently implemented, narrowly applies only to areas involving GMP and then only to a limited range of products. Some provisions have not been implemented, such as those for inspections conducted outside of the United States and the EU by EU and U.S. authorities, respectively (so-called "third-country" inspections). Those provisions should be implemented immediately. If one regulatory authority can trust the other to perform an inspection within the latter authority's own jurisdiction, the committee could find no reason to doubt the ability of the latter authority to perform a quality inspection outside its own jurisdiction—especially as these inspections are currently limited to surveillance inspections. The EU-US MRA could be expanded to go beyond its currently limited GMP focus to a broader GMP focus and to other regulatory activities, together with greater product coverage.

Recommendation 4: Regulatory authorities in the United States and the European Union (EU) should immediately implement provisions included in the current EU-US mutual recognition agreement (MRA) (e.g., those regarding so-called "third-country" good manufacturing practice [GMP] inspections). Regulatory authorities also should begin considering the potential for expanding the EU-US MRA to include reliance in areas beyond GMP and a broader scope of products under the current GMP provisions.

Facilitating Information Sharing Among International Medicines Regulators

Without a unified platform and a standard format for reporting, the sharing of assessment and inspection reports can be challenging. The committee recognizes that some regulators currently share assessment, inspection, and other reports with other regulators with whom legally authorized appropriate confidentiality arrangements exist. In instances where such arrangements do not exist, sponsors could explicitly allow regulators to share full assessment reports on specified products with specified regulators. Additionally, a recently concluded confidentiality commitment (CC) between FDA and the EU, known as the Super-CC, includes medicines. The Super-CC provides a mechanism for FDA to share essentially unredacted information with other regulatory authorities under very specific circumstances.

The committee believes that to best meet the public health goals of reliance arrangements, an opportunity exists for FDA and Congress to ensure that redaction practices optimize information sharing. The committee believes that FDA and Congress could reevaluate whether existing confidentiality restrictions are still fit-for-purpose in the 21st-century globalized environment in which medicines products exist and whether modifications are needed to meet the public health goals for these arrangements noted earlier in this report (e.g., protecting and promoting public health; reducing the burden of regulatory redundancy on patients, industry, and regulators; allowing regulators to use the finite human and financial resources they currently have most effectively and efficiently; and helping to bring needed quality medicines to patients domestically and globally as efficiently as possible).

Recommendation 5: Regulatory authorities, with guidance from their governmental leaders, should undertake determining whether current limitations on sharing regulatory work products with other regulatory authorities are still fit-for-purpose to help protect and promote public health; to reduce the burden of regulatory redundancy on patients, industry, and regulators; to allow regulators globally to best utilize the limited technical and financial resources currently available to them to meet their public health mandates; and to bring needed quality medicines to patients domestically and globally as efficiently as possible.

Evaluating Public Health Impacts of Recognition and Reliance Arrangements for Medicines

Evaluating the impacts of formal and informal recognition and reliance arrangements on public health, on the use of regulatory and industry resources, and on the essential regulatory competencies of regulatory authorities is challenging because of a dearth of frameworks, metrics, and data for use in such evaluations. The texts of existing formal and less formal recognition and reliance arrangements generally fail to incorporate review criteria or frameworks, including specific metrics, by which regulatory authorities, governments, and the broader community could evaluate the arrangements' impacts—most important, their impacts on public health. Creating a results framework with clear indicators/metrics and processes for monitoring and measuring the results of recognition and reliance arrangements could enhance understanding of their various impacts, especially on public health, and enable benefit/risk and cost/benefit analysis of formal and less formal recognition and reliance arrangements over time. Including specific evaluations of public health and other goals, metrics, and mandates in the text of future formal and less formal recognition and reliance arrangements would contribute to developing a robust body of knowledge regarding their impacts and overall utility.

Recommendation 6: When formal and informal recognition and reliance arrangements are being developed, the regulatory authorities involved should co-create a results framework with clear indicators/ metrics and processes for monitoring and measuring the arrangements' results and impacts to enhance understanding of their public health and other benefits and associated regulatory efficiencies, and enable benefit/ risk and cost/benefit analysis of the arrangements over time.

THE WAY FORWARD

As regulators and policy makers contemplate next steps, they would be wise to listen carefully to the views of patients who express their desire for effective and efficient access to quality-assured, safe, and effective medicines and advanced therapeutics that are affordable and equitably available to those who need them. Additionally, regulatory systems could be reviewed with an eye toward effectiveness (i.e., systems that do the *right thing*) and efficiency (i.e., systems that do the *thing right*). Given the human, technical, and financial resources currently available to regulatory authorities—even those that are most well-resourced—leveraging the work of other trusted authorities is essential. Eliminating redundant regulatory activities is also essential to having a system that is effective and efficient and able to meet the challenges of the globalized world, in which the products being regulated locally exist today.

At present, recognition and reliance arrangements focus on specific classes of medicines (EMA, 2019f; PIC/S, 2019a). In the future, regulatory authorities might explore the use of more agile recognition and reliance arrangements to share the ideas and perspectives of scientific experts in such areas as advanced therapeutics (e.g., gene therapy) (PIC/S, 2019b). If advanced scientific information could be shared more broadly, regulatory authorities, without local access to such information and perspectives, could also benefit from that information in deciding whether to approve such innovations within their own jurisdictions. Alternatively, regulatory authorities without local access to certain expertise, might explore the degree to which medicines approved by a trusted authority might similarly be recognized for approval in their country or region. In the end, though, regulatory authorities are responsible for regulatory decisions that affect the people in their jurisdiction. The committee believes that having a variety of different recognition and reliance arrangements from which regulators could choose would facilitate the marketing and availability of quality-assured, safe, and effective medicines necessary to safeguard the public's health.

It is the committee's view that both formal and informal recognition and reliance arrangements are important regulatory tools for helping regulatory authorities, of all resource levels, address the public health challenges posed by the increasing complexity of medicines and their globalized supply chains. The committee further contends that all medicines regulatory authorities would benefit from increased use of formal and informal recognition and reliance arrangements in conducting activities designed to fulfill their public health mission. It is the committee's view that regulation through such arrangements can now be considered a 21st-century "best regulatory practice."

1

Introduction

A quality health care system has three critical components: quality-assured practitioners, quality-assured facilities, and quality-assured health care products[1] (i.e., vaccines, pharmaceuticals, and medical devices). All three of these components must be present; if even one is absent, the system cannot provide the care patients deserve, expect, and require. It is the role of regulators to ensure that quality health care products reach the market. Moreover, although affordability and accessibility are tangential to the scope of most regulatory authorities, both are essential for ensuring a well-functioning public health system, in which quality-assured essential medicines reach those for whom they are intended.

Patients and those who work in health care expect the products they use to be what they purport to be and to work as described in the products' packaging. The fundamental issue is trust: just as patients need to be able to have confidence in the expertise of health care workers and the quality of their health care facilities, they and health workers need to be able to have confidence that the products they take and prescribe prevent or treat illness, alleviate suffering, and improve health.

A robust regulatory system that provides effective oversight of health care products throughout their lifecycle, from the laboratory to the patient, is the linchpin of product assurance. The highest priority for regulatory authorities responsible for medicines is ensuring the availability of medicines that are of high and consistent quality, safe, and effective. To this end,

[1]For quality-assured pharmaceutical health care products, this component encompasses assuring a favorable benefit/risk profile.

regulators must have access to scientifically robust, reliable data to inform their decision making. Fulfilling this mission in today's world of increasingly complex medicines that are produced in increasingly complex global manufacturing and supply chains presents significant new challenges, and meeting these challenges requires 21st-century best collaboration practices among regulatory authorities.

STUDY CONTEXT

While regulatory authorities are responsible for a wide array of health care products, this report focuses only on medicines. It does not include any discussion of medical devices, illicit drugs, naturopathic substances, or veterinary medicines, although the committee recognizes that such products are often part of the overall mandate of regulatory authorities. Moreover, this report is not designed to focus on medicines per se but to look at the regulatory authorities overseeing their quality, safety, and efficacy, and how those authorities in different jurisdictions can and do cooperate and collaborate to fulfill their responsibilities in protecting public health most effectively. These responsibilities typically involve ongoing assessment of the safety, efficacy, and manufacturing quality of all medicines, from their first introduction into human clinical trials to their widespread use following marketing authorization. The public expects not only that medicines on the market will be safe to use, work as labeled, be affordable, and be rapidly available to patients, but also that regulatory systems will make the best, most efficient use of their time and financial resources.

In the United States, the U.S. Food and Drug Administration (FDA) works hard to meet its obligations while navigating the increasing challenges and complexities associated with regulating products in a global market. Congress recognized these challenges in establishing FDA's mission by including—in addition to its public health protection mandate—a requirement that it "participate through appropriate processes with representatives of other countries to reduce the burden of regulation, harmonize regulatory requirements, and achieve appropriate reciprocal arrangements."[2] According to FDA's Center for Biologics Evaluation and Research (CBER), the agency supports this mission element through exchange mechanisms with international counterparts and organizations (FDA, 2018b). Given that medicines in the 21st century are global commodities, information exchanges have helped CBER fulfill its mandate of ensuring safe and effective medicines.

Medicines research, development, production, and distribution are decidedly global in nature and often occur in a multitude of jurisdictions

[2]Federal Food, Drug, and Cosmetic Act, 21 U.S.C. § 393.

during the lifecycle of a single product. FDA has estimated that nearly 40 percent of finished medicines/medicinal products and 80 percent of active pharmaceutical ingredients consumed by Americans are made abroad (GAO, 2016). Accordingly, regulatory authorities have had to bring a more global perspective to their work. In this global context, it has become clear that higher public health purposes and better resource utilization are best served through harmonization of technical standards and coordination of processes among regulatory authorities around the world. By sharing work and information and supporting one another through collaborative activities, regulatory authorities can bring drugs to market more quickly, avoid drug shortages, lower drug prices, communicate the risks of medicines, and become better prepared to address emerging threats. They also can optimize the use of their limited resources.

Regulatory authorities around the world have access to varying levels of resources (human, financial), but the totality of these resources is finite. Reliance allows regulatory authorities to leverage resources and expertise more efficiently. All of these relationships start with gaining knowledge of potential partners' regulatory systems and cultures, thereby building trust and confidence in their work. These relationships then evolve over time. As shown in Figure 1-1, when a regulator gains confidence in the equivalency of a counterpart's regulatory oversight, the relationship between those regulators has the potential to grow into recognition and reliance arrangements whereby one regulatory authority is willing to rely on the outputs of another. Such arrangements may start with a pilot, which often provides a safe space in which both parties can learn from each other, and in which trust is verified and built. In some instances, the trust gained during a pilot phase is enough to motivate partners to enter into more formal arrangements, the highest level of which is a mutual recognition agreement, generally agreed upon between two countries under the auspices of a trade agreement.

Many such arrangements have been implemented between well- and moderately well-resourced regulatory authorities, although lower-resourced authorities also engage in a variety of arrangements that rely on the work of other trusted authorities. A number of these collaborations (catalogued in Appendixes B and C) have the potential to enable more effective use of resources and help agencies meet the expectations of their people and their governments. By directing efforts away from duplicative inspections of low-risk manufacturers, regulatory authorities can channel more of their resources toward areas that pose greater public health challenges, including those that may stem from medicines produced and manufactured in regions with weaker regulatory oversight. In this era of globalization, moreover, strengthening and leveraging the capacities of well-resourced regulatory authorities is essential for maximal protection of global public health, as is

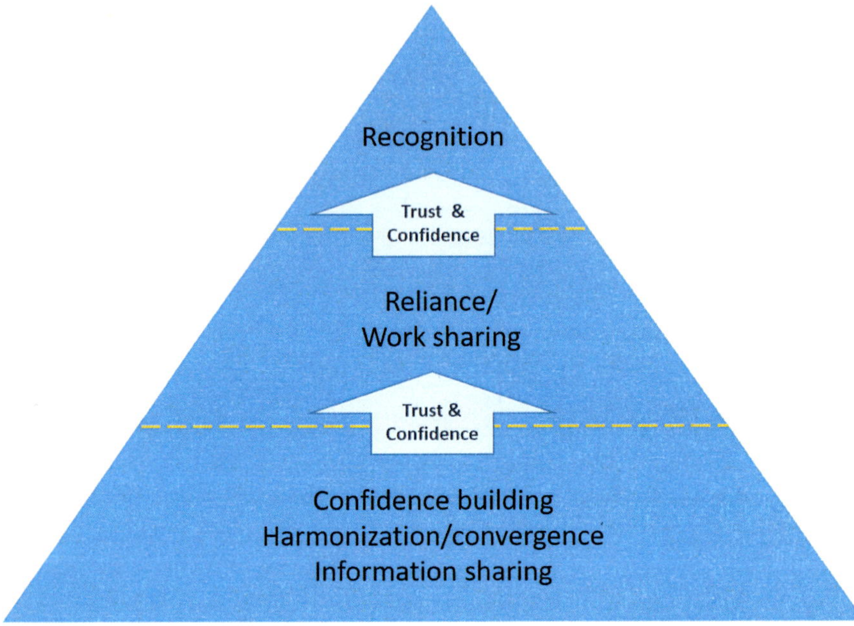

FIGURE 1-1 Building confidence and trust from and for greater reliance.
SOURCES: Adapted from a figure created by Dr. Petra Doerr, Swissmedic, and presented by Emer Cooke, World Health Organization (WHO, 2019i).

improving regulatory oversight and decision making in low-income nations. Figure 1-1 shows how trust and confidence are necessary for any form of cooperation among and between regulatory authorities, from reliance and work-sharing activities to recognition agreements (mutual and others). The arrows indicate that while confidence and trust build toward more formal arrangements, there is a certain amount of fluidity in the dotted lines for regulatory authorities to draw upon such activities as information sharing to build trust while demonstrating equivalence.

CHARGE TO THE COMMITTEE

In this context, in September 2018 FDA's Office of International Programs (now the Office of Global Policy and Strategy) charged the National Academies of Sciences, Engineering, and Medicine with convening an ad hoc committee to conduct a landscaping and analysis of mutual recognition and reliance arrangements for pharmaceutical products. The work was to include engaging relevant stakeholders in discussions that could contribute to and facilitate potential future action with respect to collaboration and cooperation among and between regulatory authorities. These discussions would include descriptions of how specific types of arrangements are or could be used, as well as the associated risks, benefits, challenges, and opportunities. The committee's report was to include a landscape of the various arrangements employed by regulatory authorities and to describe various strategies FDA and others might consider for making these arrangements even more helpful in meeting the expectations of their people and governments with respect to protecting public health and promoting quality-assured medicines (see Box 1-1 for the committee's full Statement of Task).

The committee formed to conduct this study and prepare this Consensus Study Report comprised 12 members with a broad range of expertise

BOX 1-1
Statement of Task

An ad hoc committee under the auspices of the National Academies of Sciences, Engineering, and Medicine will review and assess the use of mutual recognition/reliance agreements and informal practices of recognition/reliance, which allow regulators to use information from their counterparts at foreign drug regulatory agencies, in medicines regulation. The analysis should give particular attention to how national medicines regulatory authorities use such agreements and use such informal recognition/reliance practices and will evaluate their effects on public health, use of resources, and essential regulatory competencies. Specifically, the committee will:

- Examine the ways mutual recognition/reliance agreements and informal recognition/reliance practices are used (e.g., inspection, enforcement action, registration) including the range, scope, and time covered in the agreements. The report should discuss how all parties protect sensitive information in such arrangements;
- Discuss the benefits, risks, and challenges inherent to such agreements and informal practices, including the risks and benefits to public health. The committee should analyze how the agreements affect the efficiency and stringency of the regulatory system. Specific questions to include are whether the agreements and informal practices enable regulatory agencies to improve efficiency or redirect resources, and if so, how and what are the long-term implications for regulatory expertise as competencies evolve;
- Identify major challenges and opportunities facing national medicines regulatory authorities when implementing mutual recognition agreements; and
- Identify other regulatory areas that may lend themselves to these types of agreements and informal practices.

in areas relevant to the committee's charge, including national and international medicines regulation, law, global health policy, public health, economics, risk management, and pharmaceutical policy and manufacturing. Biographical sketches of the committee members are presented in Appendix E.

STUDY SCOPE AND APPROACH

The committee's Statement of Task drew the boundaries of the scope of this study. Because recognition and reliance arrangements have implications for virtually all countries and regulatory authorities around the globe, this report describes how different arrangements, particularly those involving regulatory authorities with higher levels of resources, could benefit the work of all regulators and provide a more universal level of quality, safety, and efficacy for medicines globally. The report touches upon but does not delve deeply into optimization efforts, including harmonization of technical standards or convergence in other appropriate areas. Nor does the report focus heavily on recognition and reliance arrangements among low-income nations. A limited discussion in these two areas is not intended to minimize the critically important harmonization work within medicines regulation, but reflects the time limitations of this study. Additionally, as noted earlier, the scope of this report is limited to medicines, encompassing both chemically and biologically based medicines and vaccines.

To address the issues raised in its Statement of Task, the committee used multiple sources in compiling the content for this report. Those sources included literature and online searches, as well as written supplemental details from regulators and information-gathering sessions involving representatives of regulatory authorities, industry, and patients. See Appendix D for a full description of the methodology used in carrying out this study.

ORGANIZATION OF THE REPORT

Following this introductory chapter, this report includes five chapters designed to respond to the Statement of Task for this study. Chapter 2 provides key background information that encompasses the issues characterizing the environment for medicines regulation, definitions of recognition and reliance, and the essential features of recognition and reliance arrangements. Chapter 3 describes how these arrangements can be viewed by policy makers and presents an overview of the regulatory functions of oversight over good manufacturing practice, batch certification, good laboratory practice, and good clinical practice. This is followed in Chapter 4 by a landscape of recognition and reliance arrangements focused on the associated challenges, benefits, and opportunities identified by stakeholder representatives who informed the committee's work, as well as the other sources noted above. Chapter 5 presents the committee's distillation of the challenges and opportunities identified in Chapter 4 as the basis for a conclusion and six recommendations, including a strategy that engages all the key stakeholders in taking action to address the key messages of this report: the importance of encouraging greater regulatory cooperation and of removing impediments that could prevent recognition and reliance arrangements from progressing. Chapter 6 closes with ideas to explore in the future, in particular, the important area of regulatory cooperation on ensuring the safety of medicines after they are available to consumers in the market.

2

The Job of Medicines Regulators in Today's World

Ensuring the health of the public through safe and effective medicines is arguably the highest priority of a medicines regulator. Carrying out this function within an increasingly complex system of production and manufacturing, alongside rapidly evolving technology and innovations in medicines, creates a whole new set of challenges and opportunities for regulators. Collaborating with others facing similar issues can be viewed as one way of managing the increasing workload faced by virtually all regulatory authorities (RAs). The key is to understand how cooperation might build coalitions by leveraging finite resources to maximize the assets of each RA. Before delving into various aspects of cooperation for the regulation of medicines, it is important to understand some of the core functions of RAs and the environment in which they now work, one that has seen unprecedented changes due primarily to advances in technology and applications stemming from the Human Genome Project (Lesko and Woodcock, 2004).

CORE FUNCTIONS OF REGULATORS AND REGULATORY AUTHORITIES

According to the World Health Organization's (WHO's) 2002 multicountry study on effective drug regulation (Ratanawijitrasin and Wondemagegnehu, 2002), the basis for regulation of medicines resides in a country's drug laws. It is up to the regulators to implement those laws—which are influenced by new developments and societal needs—by overseeing industry in the use of standards and guidelines. Key functions of regulators include "licensing, inspection of manufacturing facilities and distribution channels, product assessment and registration, adverse drug reaction monitoring, quality control, control of drug promotion and advertising, and control of clinical drug trials" (Ratanawijitrasin and Wondemagegnehu, 2002, p. 2). At times, all of these functions are carried out under a single agency, while in other instances the responsibility falls on multiple agencies, possibly at differing levels of government, which can create fragmentation and decrease the effectiveness of regulation. Some RAs are given functions, such as drug manufacturing and procurement, that would be viewed as conflicts of interest with the agency's mission of drug regulation. This situation speaks to the issue of financing. Most RAs are financed through a mix of government support and user fees, while a small number of RAs are entirely dependent on user fees. The financial structure of an agency, according to the WHO report, should not influence regulatory decisions; however, RAs with inadequate staff, poor working conditions, or poor financing may be subject to compromise (Babigumira et al., 2018).

REGULATORS WORKING TOGETHER

Most, if not all, well- and moderately well-resourced RAs have shifted to a risk-based approach to regulation. For each of them, this includes allocating regulatory resources more proportionately so that, for example, manufacturers of medicines with greater risk are inspected more frequently than those that present a much lower risk. The approach also includes working together with other RAs. Those with similar structures, functions, and national characteristics might find a more natural fit for working together, depending on the collaborative activity undertaken. Such activities can be divided into pre- and post-marketing efforts (Babigumira et al., 2018). Pre-marketing activities, as outlined in the U.S. Agency for International Development's 2018 Risk-Based Resource Allocation Framework (Babigumira et al., 2018), include licensing of premises and persons, inspection, evaluation and registration, and quality control testing. Quality control testing can also occur post-marketing along with product quality monitoring and surveillance, safety/pharmacovigilance, and enforcement of pharmaceutical laws and regulations.

Good Regulatory Practices for Cooperation

The Organisation for Economic Co-operation and Development (OECD) describes good regulatory outcomes as "almost always a cooperative effort: by the regulator and other regulators, the regulated, and often the broader community" (OECD, 2014, p. 5). OECD notes further that governance arrangements can foster cooperative efforts and outlines areas of good governance for regulators that could lay a foundation for strong cooperation and collaboration. Six of these areas are:

1. role clarity—functions are clear and without conflicts;
2. preventing undue influence and maintaining trust—objective, impartial, consistent decision making;
3. accountability and transparency—accountable to government and the public;
4. engagement—enhance and maintain public and stakeholder confidence;
5. funding—protect independence but be transparent to heighten confidence in decisions; and
6. performance evaluation—to understand impacts of own actions and drive improvements.

WHO is developing guidelines for good regulatory practices for RAs specific to medicines. While this and another WHO effort on good reliance practices remain works in progress, there does appear to be potential overlap between the two concepts whereby good regulatory practice involves reliance. WHO's draft of the guidelines for good regulatory practice states that, "regulations should include sufficient administrative flexibility to allow for participation in international cooperation frameworks, such as for information-sharing, convergence, harmonization, work-sharing, reliance and recognition" (WHO, 2016b, p. 10).

RECOGNITION AND RELIANCE

As part of its benchmarking tool, WHO (2018b) defines recognition as the routine acceptance of another RA's—or other trusted institution's—regulatory decisions based on the work products of that other agency. In contrast, reliance is defined as being more flexible, giving an RA in one jurisdiction the option of taking into account work products (e.g., inspection reports, scientific assessment reports, joint assessment reports produced together with another RA) of another authority or trusted institution in reaching its own decision. These definitions are presented in Box 2-1. A decision to *routinely accept* or to *take into account* the work of another regulator is the choice of the reliant RA and might be based on a variety of factors including the context in which a decision is being made, access to resources, and whether there is sufficient trust and confidence in the RA being relied on for information. But regardless of whether an RA uses recognition or reliance, in the end it is the responsibly of the RA to protect the health of its people and thus make the best regulatory decisions for its country. In this regard (illustrated in Figure 2-1), recognition can be viewed

BOX 2-1
World Health Organization (WHO)
Definitions of Recognition and Reliance

Recognition: The routine acceptance by the regulatory authority (RA) in one jurisdiction of the work products* and regulatory decisions of another RA or other trusted institution. Recognition indicates that evidence of conformity with the regulatory requirements of country A is sufficient to meet the regulatory requirements of country B. Recognition may be unilateral, bilateral, or multilateral, although recognition is usually manifested as the subject of mutual recognition agreements.

Reliance: The act whereby the regulatory authority in one jurisdiction may take into account and give significant weight to (i.e., totally or partially rely on work products by) another regulatory authority or trusted institution in reaching its own decision. The relying authority remains responsible and accountable for decisions taken, even when it relies on the decisions and information of others.

SOURCE: Adapted from WHO, 2018b.

*The committee uses the term "work product" to describe the full spectrum of good practices products of RAs.

as a subset, or a more stringent form of reliance, with the mutual recognition agreement (MRA) as the most stringent form of all.

Recognition and Reliance Among Well- and Lower-Resourced Regulatory Authorities

The way in which an RA views recognition and reliance may have more to do with how well-resourced that agency is in relation to another RA. For example, equally well-resourced RAs would typically take a horizontal perspective in sharing information rather than the more unidirectional approach that would likely result from lower-resourced RAs relying on the work of well-resourced or moderately well-resourced RAs. These concepts are explained in greater detail below.

Recognition and Reliance Among Well-Resourced Regulatory Authorities

In the case of recognition and reliance between well-resourced RAs, it is necessary for technical regulatory requirements as well as procedures in inspection/review of medicines manufacturers to be fairly close, if not identical. If a good manufacturing practice (GMP) itself is different between

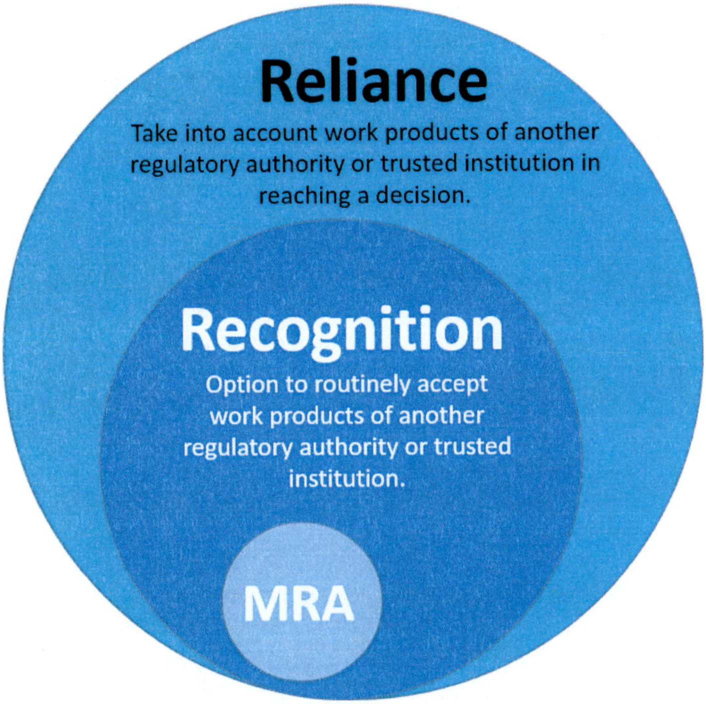
Reliance
Take into account work products of another regulatory authority or trusted institution in reaching a decision.
Recognition
Option to routinely accept work products of another regulatory authority or trusted institution.
MRA

FIGURE 2-1 Recognition as a subset of reliance.
SOURCES: Adapted from a figure created by Dr. Petra Doerr, Swissmedic, and presented by Emer Cooke, World Health Organization (WHO, 2019i).

country A and country B, joint inspections, regardless of how many times they may be conducted, cannot facilitate reliance on the inspection results. Because RAs involved in horizontal recognition and reliance arrangements are of similar or comparable capacities, the collaboration is usually mutual and "trust" here means that one agency has concluded that the other does as good a job as its own reviewers or inspectors.

Recognition and Reliance Among Lower-Resourced Regulatory Authorities

A lower-resourced RA can base its decisions on the work products of well-resourced, trusted RAs. The extent to which the reliance occurs can vary from critically examining inspection reports or reviews and potentially reaching different conclusions to accepting other agencies' decisions without further examination. This type of recognition and reliance would not typically be considered mutual, and in such cases, regulations need not be completely harmonized between the relying and the relied-on RAs. The "trust" here is from lower-resourced to well-resourced or moderately well-resourced RAs. Trust in these instances can be formed without such critical examination of the capabilities of the RA being relied on as is necessary for horizontal recognition and reliance, and can be naturally reputation-based because of the resource constraint involved. Such recognition and reliance apply to regulatory oversight during the pre- and post-approval phases. An example is the Caribbean Regulatory System (CRS), where numerous small states make up the Caribbean Community. Each state lacks the resources and capacity necessary to fully conduct medicines regulation on its own so the CRS uses a regional reliance mechanism—relying on trusted RAs within the Pan American Health Organization, the European Union (EU), and WHO prequalification—to help inform its decisions about which medicines to recommend for regional market authorization (PAHO, 2019b).

Trust as a Foundational Element

What underlies all recognition and reliance arrangements is trust. Medicines RAs cannot rely if they do not trust the provenance and findings of another RA. This means there are necessary early steps in building trust that, over time, can grow stronger through using common international standards (harmonization) and report formats, and through working together. Figure 2-2 illustrates trust in the regulatory sense and how it forms the backbone of any reliance process. Prior to executing formal reliance arrangements, RAs will likely need to pilot an established process of joint inspections/working together and even auditing of each other's work. All of these efforts build confidence in the systems and procedures of the respective RAs. In contrast, other forms of reliance exist that take a more unidirectional approach to the medicines approval process by fully embracing the results of trusted RAs.

COOPERATION AND COLLABORATION TOOLS OF REGULATORY AUTHORITIES

Different tools are available for recognition and reliance across the product lifecycle. These are collectively referred to in this report as "arrangements." Arrangements can be formal agreements put in place, for example, through Memoranda of Understanding (MOUs), confidentiality commitments, and MRAs; or they can be informal through the establishment of ad hoc committees, working parties, and other, more topic-specific working groups (EMA, 2019g). WHO's draft guidelines for good regulatory practice note that "less formal practices include sharing of information, scientific

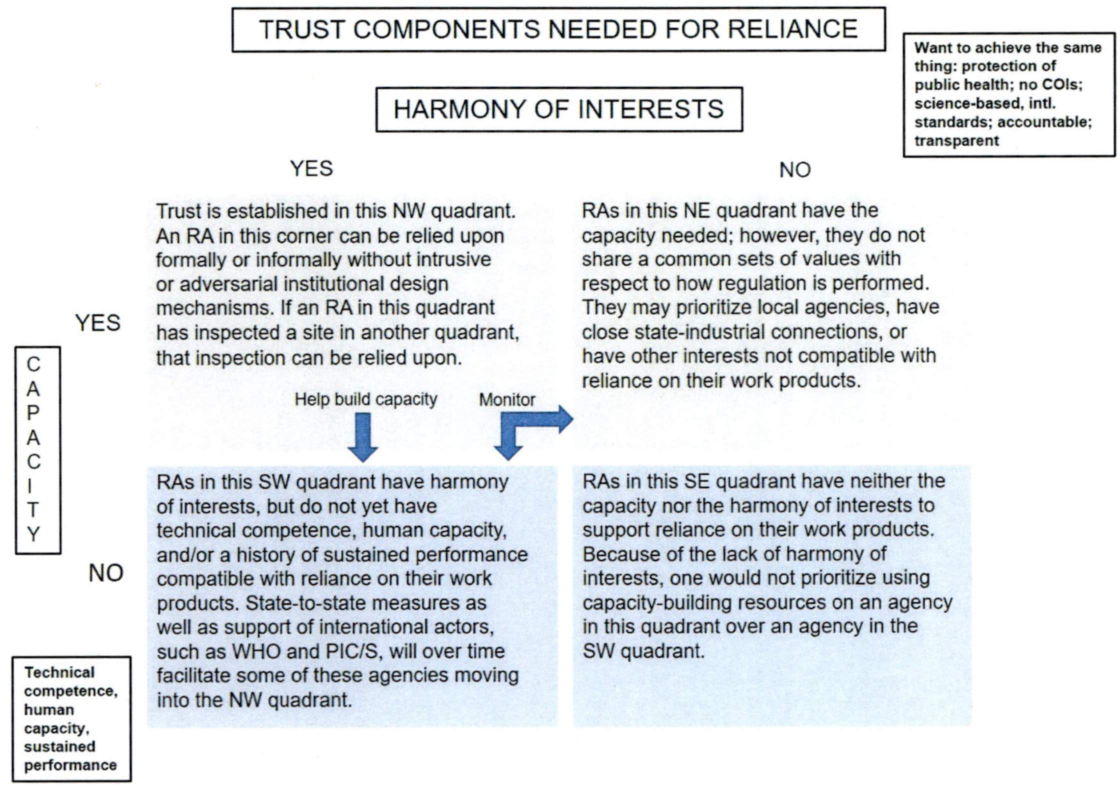

FIGURE 2-2 Trust components needed for reliance.
NOTE: COI = conflict of interest; PIC/S = Pharmaceutical Inspection Co-operation Scheme; RA = regulatory authority; WHO = World Health Organization.

collaboration, common risk assessment, joint reviews, and development of standards" (WHO, 2016b, p. 27). Some formal collaborative activities include what might be considered less formal interactions through regularly scheduled calls and meetings that build trust between regulators as they move toward greater confidence levels for reliance.

In many cases, pilot activities can be set up under the formal mechanism of confidential arrangements (also known as confidentiality commitments) between RAs. The arrangements differ, but generally speaking, they allow regulators to exchange confidential information that is not in the public domain. Pilots can be useful tools for building trust and confidence between regulators from different jurisdictions. One example is the International Generic Drug Regulators Pilot that began in 2012 as a collaborative arrangement among RAs from Australia, Canada, Chinese Taipei, the EU, and Switzerland (EMA, 2015). It was modeled on the EU system, which is a network of 50 RAs from 31 countries (28 Member States, Iceland, Liechtenstein, and Norway) that rely on each other through application of the mutual recognition principle and common regulations and procedures. Another example of a work-sharing arrangement (described in Box 2-2) is the Australia-Canada-Singapore-Switzerland (ACSS) Consortium. It started in 2007 as a pilot to maximize international cooperation and is now exploring opportunities for information and work sharing in such areas as:

BOX 2-2
Work Sharing:
Australia-Canada-Singapore-Switzerland (ACSS) Consortium

The ACSS Consortium is a collaborative initiative of like-minded medium-sized regulatory authorities (Australia's Therapeutic Goods Administration [TGA], Health Canada, Singapore's Health Sciences Authority, and the Swiss Agency for Therapeutic Products) that collaborate during the marketing authorization review of new drugs. Regulatory authorities face similar challenges, such as increasing workload and the growing complexity of the medicinal applications being regulated, which contribute to increasing pressure on available resources. The purpose of this consortium is to build synergies and share knowledge among these four regulatory authorities, thereby enhancing the efficiency of their individual regulatory systems. Work sharing in the marketing authorization of new medicines is one of the initiatives of the ACSS Consortium. Apalutamide (Erlyand®, Erleada®) was the first medicine registered that had been evaluated under the ACSS Consortium's New Chemical Entities Work Sharing initiative. The review also utilized TGA's new priority review pathway.

SOURCES: HC, 2018; TGA, 2019a.

- generic medicines registration,
- assessment reports for new prescription medicines,
- information sharing and investigations into post-market medicine safety,
- alignment of information technology systems for information sharing, and
- development of technical guidelines (TGA, 2019b).

MOUs are another tool frequently used by RAs to coordinate activities and share information. They are nonbinding agreements that can vary greatly in their scope depending on their purpose and the parties involved. Often, MOUs allow RAs a more formal route to clarifying the roles and responsibilities of the parties. A Memorandum of Cooperation (MOC) is similar to an MOU in that it is not legally binding. This tool has been used by Japan to set guidelines for cooperation between parties. Unlike MOUs and MOCs, recognition agreements can be legally binding.

Mutual Recognition Agreements

While reliance arrangements promote the sharing of information and facilitate fewer redundant inspections and other regulatory activities, MRAs allow agencies not just to rely on each other's work products but also to recognize them as equal to the work of their own reviewers or inspectors. For the EU, MRAs allow for reliance on the GMP inspection systems of other RAs, information sharing based on inspections and quality, and the waiving of batch testing of those products imported into EU territories. It should be noted that while safeguarding the public's health is intrinsic to MRAs, they are in the end "trade agreements that aim to facilitate market access" (EMA, 2019f). As such, they tend to be laborious to develop and negotiate and are labor-intensive to maintain; however, the required preparation and maintenance work is often deemed worthwhile as it prevents duplication of effort, makes precious resources available, and expedites approval time and market release, all of which are of great public health benefit. As is shown in later chapters of this report, these benefits are also achieved through the use of reliance arrangements that do not pose many of the challenges associated with MRAs. See Appendix B for a list of the MRAs that are a primary focus of this report.

Unilateral and Multilateral Recognition

Unilateral recognition allows one RA's decisions to be informed partially or fully by the work of another. Some Latin American countries take such an approach. One example is Mexico's RA, Comisión Federal para la Protección contra Riesgos Sanitarios (COFEPRIS), which in 2012 established a unilateral agreement with the EU to use work carried out at the European Medicines Agency (EMA) during its single marketing authorization process (WHO, 2016a). COFEPRIS set up other similar unilateral processes with the U.S. Food and Drug Administration (FDA), Health Canada, Australia's Therapeutic Goods Administration (TGA), and Swissmedic to expedite the approval of new medicines and their entry onto the Mexican market (Patel et al., 2019). It appears that other Latin American countries (i.e., Argentina, Dominican Republic, Ecuador, El Salvador, Paraguay, Peru, and Uruguay) may also use unilateral approaches based on information from what the countries deem to be trusted sources (Sravani et al., 2017). With this arrangement, those countries that are relied on are placed in a position whereby approval decisions in their jurisdiction have relevance and impacts beyond their own country or region.

The European Economic Area (EEA), composed of Iceland, Liechtenstein, and Norway, has MRAs with Australia, Canada, New Zealand, and Switzerland on GMP (and additionally, on good laboratory practice in the MRA between EEA and the European Free Trade Association/Switzerland) that are modeled on the EU MRAs. Another example is the mutual recognition arrangements of the Association of Southeast Asian Nations (ASEAN) Member States. In this case, all ASEAN member states are "obliged to recognize and accept the [GMP] inspection reports and certificates issued by ASEAN Inspection Services without duplicating GMP inspection in each other's territory" (HSA, n.d.). COFEPRIS also has multilateral agreements with a number of regional and international organizations, with different scopes for different conformity assessment bodies (La Entidad Mexicana de la Acreditación, 2019).

Cooperation Through Harmonization

Broader efforts among countries for cooperation on aspects of the regulation of medicines have taken place under the auspices of regulatory harmonization (APEC, 2019; ICH, 2019; IPRP, 2019; PAHO, 2019a). Regulatory reliance may be facilitated by having RAs converge more than diverge on such matters as procedures and common formats for reports and forms, as appropriate, and as supported by international organizations such as the International Council for Harmonisation of Technical Requirements for Pharmaceuticals for Human Use, and by bringing regulators together for various collaborative and cooperative efforts (see Box 2-3 for a summary of harmonization, convergence, and reliance efforts through international organizations).

BOX 2-3
Representative Multilateral, International Cooperative and Collaborative Efforts in Pharmaceutical Regulation

- **International Council for Harmonisation of Technical Requirements for Pharmaceuticals for Human Use (ICH):** ICH brings together the major regulatory authorities and the pharmaceutical industry to discuss scientific and technical aspects of drug registration. Since its inception in 1990, ICH has gradually evolved to respond to the increasingly global nature of drug development by preparing numerous harmonized technical requirements for authorization and regulatory oversight of pharmaceuticals for human use.*
- **International Pharmaceutical Regulators Programme (IPRP):** IPRP was created to establish a forum for its regulatory members and observers to exchange information on issues of mutual interest and enable regulatory cooperation. This venue assists in maximizing potential efficiencies in addressing the increasingly complex global regulatory environment, facilitates the implementation of ICH and other internationally harmonized technical guidelines for pharmaceuticals for human use, promotes collaboration and regulatory convergence, and contributes to the coordination of international efforts related to regulation of medicinal products for human use.
- **International Coalition of Medicines Regulatory Authorities (ICMRA):** ICMRA is a voluntary, executive-level, strategic coordinating, advocacy and leadership entity of regulatory authorities that work together to address current and emerging human medicine regulatory and safety challenges globally, provide direction for areas and activities common to many regulatory authorities' missions, identify areas for potential synergies, and wherever possible, leverage existing initiatives/enablers and resources. ICMRA will provide a global architecture to support enhanced communication, information sharing, and crisis response and address regulatory science issues.
- **International Conference of Drug Regulatory Authorities (ICDRA):** The conferences have been held since 1980 to provide drug regulatory authorities of all 194 World Health Organization (WHO) Member States with a forum to meet and discuss priorities for action in national and international regulation of medicines, vaccines, biomedicines, and herbals. ICDRA's aim is to promote the exchange of information and collaborative approaches to issues of common concern, and find ways to strengthen collaboration and serve as a tool for WHO and drug regulatory authorities in their efforts to harmonize regulation and improve the safety, efficacy, and quality of medicines.
- **Pharmaceutical Inspection Co-operation Scheme (PIC/S):** PIC/S is a non-binding, informal cooperative arrangement among regulatory authorities in the area of good manufacturing practice (GMP) for medicinal products for human or veterinary use. It has 52 participating authorities and is open to any authority having a comparable GMP inspection system and aiming to harmonize inspection procedures and standards and facilitate cooperation and networking among competent authorities and regional and international organizations, thus increasing mutual confidence.

continued

BOX 2-3 Continued

- **Australia-Canada-Singapore-Switzerland (ACSS) Consortium:** The ACSS Consortium is a coalition, formed in 2007 by "like-minded" regulatory authorities to promote information and work sharing. Its goal is to reduce duplication and increase each agency's capacity to ensure that consumers have timely access to high-quality, safe, and effective therapeutic products.

SOURCES: ICH, 2019; ICMRA, 2019; IPRP, 2019; PIC/S, 2019c; TGA, 2019b; WHO, 2019h.

*Veterinary ICH (VICH) also exists, but it is a different organization with its secretariat role fulfilled by HealthforAnimals. VICH is a trilateral (European Union [EU]–Japan–United States) program, involving several observer organizations, aimed at harmonizing technical requirements for veterinary product registration. Its full title is the International Cooperation on Harmonisation of Technical Requirements for Registration of Veterinary Medicinal Products. VICH was officially launched in April 1996 (VICH, 2019).

Strengthening Regulatory Systems for Medicines Through Transparency

RAs in low- and middle-income countries face multiple challenges that vary by country. According to Roth and colleagues (2018), these challenges tend to include access to medicines—in part because of limited commercial returns for industry—as well as access to evidence-based data, both pre- and post-market. In some instances, donor organizations, the pharmaceutical industry, and public–private partnerships have attempted to improve the supply of medicines in developing countries, but despite these efforts, a lag time persists. Typically, it takes 4 to 7 years between initial approval by one RA (generally in a developed country) and final approval (in the developing country) (Ahonkhai et al., 2016). Numerous reasons were suggested for the delay, including "failure to leverage or rely on the findings from reviews already performed by competent regulatory authorities, disparate requirements for product approval by the countries, and lengthy timelines by manufacturers to respond to regulatory queries" (Ahonkhai et al., 2016, p. 1).

Some efforts are under way to build regulatory capacity for accelerated registration through WHO prequalification (WHO, 2019c) and the work of the International Coalition of Medicines Regulatory Authorities in the area of GMP (ICMRA, 2017). As capacity is built within some RAs to better utilize information from trusted authorities, fuller access to information, reports, and data will likely become more valuable. In an effort to promote greater openness and transparency, WHO, EMA, and FDA have sought to make some information publicly available (EMA, 2019b; FDA, 2015b; WHO, 2019d). These reports exclude confidential proprietary information, and in the case of WHO, are posted only on its website with the manufacturer's approval. Similarly, openness between well-resourced and lower-resourced RAs would almost certainly require input from industry.

3

What Policy Makers Need to Know About Today's Regulatory Environment

In understanding the current regulatory environment, it is important to recognize the growing complexity of medicines research and development, production, and manufacturing. In many instances, manufacturing of medicines has become a global endeavor crossing multiple national borders before a product is distributed to numerous local markets around the world. Not only have supply chains grown in complexity, but medicines themselves have also become more complex, both biologically and chemically. Figure 3-1 shows the range of medicines, from the simplest products with well-defined chemical structures, to highly complicated gene or cell therapies using extremely advanced drug research, development, and manufacturing methodologies. Of note is that as medicines go from simple to complex, regulatory oversight will follow a similar path. However, not all regulatory authorities have the resources to train or hire those with the requisite skillset to assess more complex products for approval or to monitor their safety post-approval (Luigetti et al., 2016). Cooperation and collaboration in their many forms represent tools regulatory authorities can use to overcome resource constraints, avoid duplication of efforts, and leverage expertise across borders for improved decision making within a local jurisdiction or region. All of these tools fit under the umbrella of recognition and reliance arrangements.

OVERVIEW OF GOOD PRACTICES

It is industry's responsibility to comply with rules and scientific and technical standards established for products, and it is the regulator's respon-

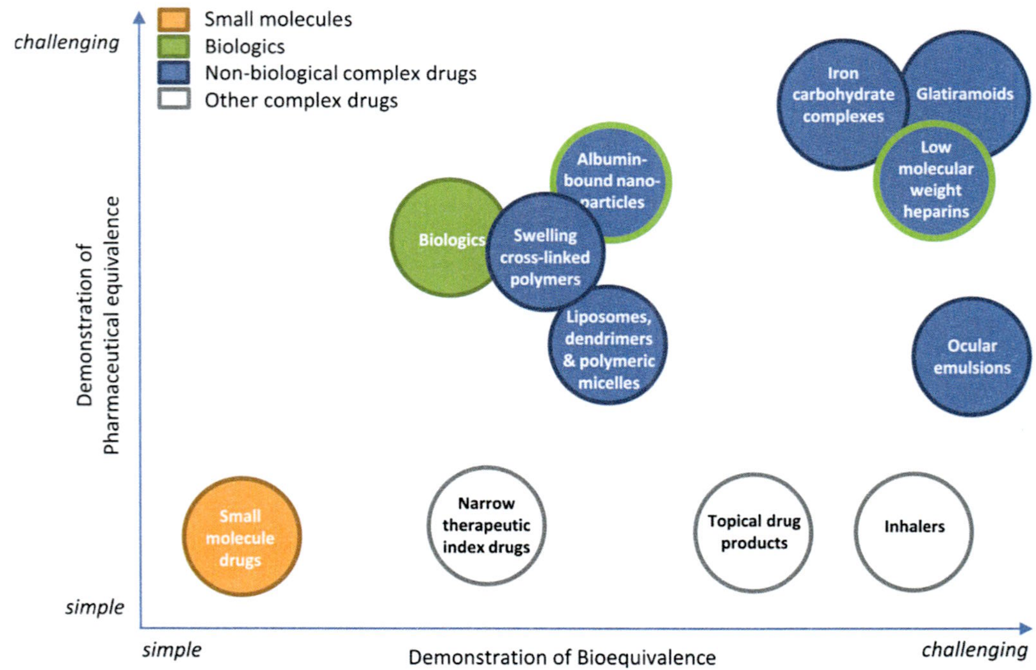

FIGURE 3-1 The complex drug landscape.
NOTES: Drug products are positioned on the basis of the challenge to assess the pharmaceutical equivalence (PE) and bioequivalence (BE) of two drug products (i.e., the reference product and its generic version). The percentage of new medicines categorized as "complex" is increasing. From a global perspective, the resources and expertise needed to assess the expanding number of complex medicines are limited. Complete execution of recognition and reliance arrangements will be essential if regulatory authorities plan to assess the broad spectrum of medicines being manufactured in a timely and reliable way.
SOURCE: Hussaarts et al., 2017.

sibility to oversee compliance with these rules and standards (Rönninger et al., 2012) and to work with the larger community to develop new standards as technology and scientific knowledge improve. For medicines, there are regulations describing compliance activities and good practices across the lifecycle of a medicine from preclinical research to post-marketing surveillance. Guidance is provided by regulatory authorities at each stage (as shown in Figure 3-2), but it is up to industry to interpret that guidance and apply it to their situation. Good laboratory practice (GLP) sets guidelines for ensuring that laboratory data are of high quality and reliable in the preclinical phase, good clinical practice (GCP) guides aspects of studies involving human subjects, good manufacturing practice (GMP) provides guidance for the manufacturing, production and distribution of medicines, and good pharmacovigilance practice provides guidance for the appropriate oversight of products once they have been released onto the general market. Assuring an overall positive benefit/risk profile to the most appropriate level possible is essential throughout the entire medicine product lifecycle.

In this report, regulatory work products—administrative documents produced by a regulator as a result of a regulatory authority's evaluation—are differentiated from medical products that include but are not limited to medicines. These work products might include an inspection report or certificate of compliance for GMP, official batch release, or an assessment report regarding the evaluation of the clinical and statistical elements of the product clinical dataset used in the application requesting approval to market a new medicine.

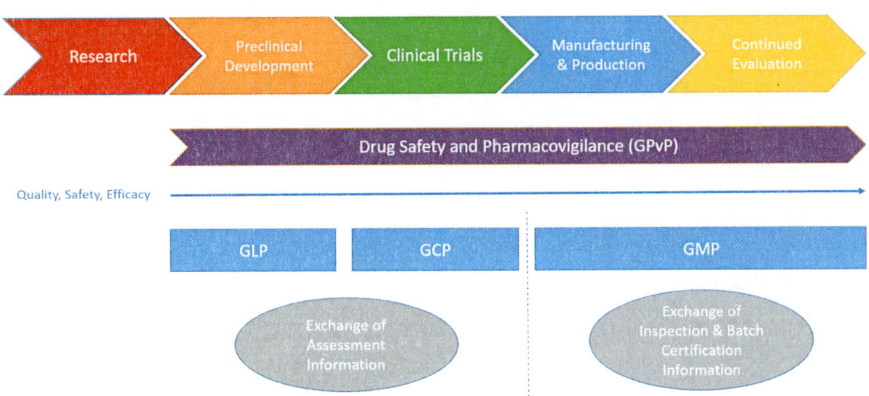

FIGURE 3-2 Lifecycle of a medicine.

Good Manufacturing Practice

All current mutual recognition agreements (MRAs) regarding the regulation of medicines include provisions for relying on a partner for GMP inspections. Each MRA, with the exception of that between the United States and the European Union (EU), is based primarily on the exchange of GMP certificates (see Table 3-1), with the provision of inspection reports upon request (the U.S. Food and Drug Administration [FDA] does not issue GMP certificates in practice). Inspections covered under each of the MRAs are intended to confirm that the products are manufactured in compliance with current agreed-upon GMP. Of note is that none of the current MRAs include provisions for GMPs for advanced therapy medicinal products, although this may be an area of future interest between the United States and the EU.

Before countries sign MRAs, their regulatory authorities spend a significant amount of time evaluating each other's systems and procedures to attain a level of confidence in each other's output. In addition, one condition of an MRA or any reliance agreement is the conclusion that all

TABLE 3-1 Comparison of MRAs

Instrument Used for Information Exchange Between Manufacturer and Importer and Between Mutual Recognition Agreement (MRA) Partners				
MRA	Batch Testing	Good Manufacturing Practice (GMP) Certificate	Rapid Alert	Inspection Report
EU-AUS	Yes	Yes	Yes	No
EU-NZ	Yes	Yes	Yes	No
EU-CH	Yes	Yes	Yes	No
EU-CAN	Yes	Yes	Yes	No
EU-JAPAN	Yes	Yes	Yes	No
EU-ISRAEL	Yes	Yes	Yes	No
EU-US	Yes for EU	No	Yes	Yes
Australia-New Zealand	Yes	Yes	Yes*	No
Australia-Canada	Yes	Yes	Yes	No
Australia-Singapore	Yes	Yes	Yes	No
Canada-Switzerland	Yes	Yes	Yes	No

NOTES: See Appendix B for a fuller description. Aus = Australia; CAN = Canada; CH = Switzerland; EU = European Union; NZ = New Zealand; US = United States.

*Rapid alert system not designated in MRA, but executed through Pharmaceutical Inspection Co-operation Scheme (PIC/S) membership.

SOURCES: Adapted from Saint-Raymond, 2019; EU-US MRA.

authorities involved are "capable" of evaluating GMP and taking appropriate actions when a facility is out of compliance. These evaluation activities foster trust and confidence. While MRAs are established on both a foundation of trust and years of cross-evaluation, each regulatory authority is ultimately responsible for the health of its population. As a result, under specified conditions, MRAs contain clauses stating that each party has the right to conduct an inspection in any facility even if a partner regulatory authority has already done so. At the time MRAs are established, procedures for communicating noncompliance findings to partner authorities are outlined. Each regulatory authority retains sovereignty and is responsible for interpreting inspection results. It is a regulatory authority's privilege and responsibility to ask questions and take enforcement action if there is reason to believe that a manufacturer's practices have compromised the quality of a product or are likely to do so, thereby compromising the health of that regulator's population.

FDA defines enforcement as "action taken by an authority to protect the public from products of suspect quality, safety, and effectiveness or to assure that products are manufactured in compliance with appropriate laws, regulations, standards, and commitments made as part of the approval to market a product."[1] Common enforcement actions are a request for voluntary compliance, suspension of product distribution, detention at the border of the importing country, recall or withdrawal of the batch(es), and requests for additional information or inspections.[2] Similarly, Health Canada has MRAs with the EU, Switzerland, and the European Economic Area (EEA). Health Canada's enforcement actions in response to GMP noncompliance are similar to those of FDA and include, but are not limited to, written correspondence and requests for plans for corrective measures and/or additional assessments, public advisories, removal, and seizure and/or destruction of existing products.

Rather than providing specific details regarding the use of enforcement actions within the agreement, most MRAs make reference to the importance of honoring each party's established regulatory commitments to quality, safety, and public health. Each regulatory authority can take enforcement actions it deems appropriate. Under MRAs, partner regulatory authorities are not required to take the same enforcement actions in response to an inspection report; however, given the MRA precondition of regulatory authority equivalence, authorities in an MRA are expected to take enforcement actions that are congruent with and imply similar reactions to noncompliant practices. At the same time, it should be understood that action taken to suspend manufacturing activities at a site in

[1]21 CFR § 26.1.
[2]21 CFR § 26.21.

an MRA partner's own territory will directly impact supply to other territories, including MRA partners, without any direct intervention by the other authority. The MRA between Australia and Singapore highlights the independent authority of each party to "determine the level of protection it considers necessary with regard to health, safety, and the environment"; consequently, neither party is bound by contract to take the same enforcement actions as the other. Regardless of the actions either party takes, both have agreed to notify the other regulatory authority of any enforcement actions within 15 days.

Batch Certificate

While all MRAs are designed to minimize duplicative inspections of manufacturing sites of similar interest between the signatories, virtually all existing MRAs go further by waiving batch testing in the importing country (see Box 3-1). A batch certificate can be issued confirming that each individual batch (fully finished or partially manufactured) has been manufactured and checked in compliance with the appropriate laws, marketing authorization requirements, and GMP. The certificate is normally issued by the exporting manufacturer and may, if necessary, be validated or even issued by the competent regulatory authority of the exporting country (WHO, 2019f).

Some MRAs provide for acknowledging testing done by official laboratories or batch disposition decisions for certain types of products (e.g., blood products, some vaccines). At present, however, the scope of the EU-US MRA does not include regulatory activities associated with these product types, although it contains a provision for waiving batch testing for those medicines covered under the MRA. Having an MRA or other agreement that facilitates waiving batch testing in the importing country or mutually recognizes official batch testing reduces costs and product wastage and allows importers and regulatory authorities to redirect resources toward areas of greater risk instead of performing redundant regulatory laboratory testing (Garbe et al., 2015).

Good Laboratory Practice

GLP in the pharmaceutical industry is often guided by multiple resources, including a handbook from the World Health Organization (WHO, 2009), rules established by FDA for nonclinical laboratory studies,[3] and principles set forth by the Organisation for Economic Co-operation and Development (OECD). These combined resources help set the boundaries for nonclinical

[3]21 CFR Part 58.

BOX 3-1
Batch Release

Batch testing is only a small part of the batch release process, but mutual recognition agreements (MRAs) make the process more efficient. "'Qualified Persons' in the European Union (EU) Member States need not batch test human medicines covered by the EU-US MRA provided they have verified that these controls have been carried out in the United States for products manufactured in and imported from the United States" (EMA, 2019f). The U.S. manufacturer provides the "Qualified Person" of the EU importer with a batch certificate to this effect.

For certain vaccines and blood products imported into the EU from Switzerland, there is no need to submit samples to an EU Official Laboratory if a batch release certificate (not to be confused with the batch certificate referred to above) has already been issued by the Swiss Official Medicines Control Laboratory for the batch in question and vice versa. Vaccines and blood products are currently not within the scope of the EU-US MRA.

Ultimately, the decision to release any batch of product onto the EU market rests with the EU manufacturer or importer, and release can take place only after a "Qualified Person" has certified the batch in question (the batch certificate in this case can be similar to the one recommended for use under an MRA). MRAs do not alter this requirement.

SOURCES: EMA, 2019f; EudraLex, Volume 4, EU Guidelines for Good Manufacturing Practice for Medicinal Products for Human and Veterinary Use, Annex 16: Certification by a Qualified Person and Batch Release.

testing conducted prior to the approval of a medicinal product through strict guidelines for generating quality-assured and reliable test data while using an environmentally safe and animal numbers reduction approach (OECD, 2019). Regulators are allowed to rely on certifications and inspections provided for GLP under some MRAs (e.g., EU-Japan; Switzerland-Canada, Switzerland-EU; Switzerland-EEA, which includes Norway, Iceland, and Liechtenstein [see Appendix B]). According to OECD, significant cost savings to industry and governments are possible through mutual acceptance of such laboratory data. Part of OECD's estimated €309 million total savings each year (from all sectors) includes a reduction in the number of animals used for testing purposes (OECD, 2019).

In addition to GLP covered under MRAs, the United States and the Netherlands entered into a Memorandum of Understanding (MOU) under their confidentiality arrangement that reciprocally recognizes both countries' GLP programs (FDA, 1988). This MOU was signed only after comparable standards of GLP had been established by the respective national authorities. As part of the agreement, both parties are required to regularly communicate and share information and data unrelated to trade secrets or confidential commercial or financial disclosures.

The International Laboratory Accreditation Cooperation (ILAC) recognition arrangement links accrediting bodies around the world through a peer review system that includes a review of the impartiality and consistency of those performing inspections (ILAC, 2019). While ILAC signatories are not regulators, the program does call to light the importance of the International Organization for Standardization/International Electrotechnical Commission 17020:2012 requirements for establishing the competence of bodies performing inspections as a foundation for sharing in the area of GLP (ISO, 2012).

Good Clinical Practice

The International Council for Harmonisation of Technical Requirements for Pharmaceuticals for Human Use has published a GCP guideline (ICH E6 R1) for clinical trials involving human subjects (ICH, 2016). This guideline, agreed upon initially in 1996, establishes ethical and scientific standards for ensuring the safety and privacy of clinical trial participants and the credibility of data on trial results. The most recent addendum to the publication provides a "unified standard for the EU, Japan, the US, Canada, and Switzerland to facilitate the mutual acceptance of data from clinical trials by the regulatory authorities in these jurisdictions" (ICH, 2016, p. 1).

The European Medicines Agency (EMA) and FDA Good Clinical Practice Initiative that commenced after an 18-month pilot test between 2009 and 2011 involved sharing information on clinical trial site inspections, as well as collaborating on inspections (EMA, 2011). As with similar efforts, as discussed in Chapter 2, confidence and trust are built between partner regulatory agencies during the pilot phases of such initiatives. Thus, while GCP is not part of the recently functional EU-US MRA for pharmaceuticals, it is possible that the associated regulatory authorities could move beyond trust building and knowledge sharing and agree to expand the operational scope of the MRA to include recognition of each other's GCP inspections of clinical trials. Doing so could help repurpose both agencies' finite human and financial inspection resources.

Confidentiality Arrangements

Confidentiality arrangements are often what allow regulatory bodies to enter into cooperative arrangements such as the EU-US initiative. Confidentiality arrangements allow parties to exchange confidential information, although they are not a prerequisite for building trust and knowledge between regulators. For example, the GCP Inspectors Working Group meets four times per year at EMA. The group includes representatives from the GCP inspectorates of the EEA Member States, as well as observers from candidate countries and Switzerland (EMA, 2013). In addition to the Working Group, WHO is invited to participate in these meetings. The Working Group's regular interactions provide a forum for strengthening relationships among the peer groups from the regulatory authorities.

Because of the large number of redactions common with FDA inspection and assessment reports, a "super confidentiality commitment" (Super-CC) was established between the United States and the EU designed to minimize redactions, thereby making the reports more usable. The authority for FDA to enter into such super confidentiality arrangements under certain conditions is a specific provision added to U.S. law in the past few years.

PUBLIC HEALTH MANDATE

Part of the responsibility of national regulators in protecting the public's health when relying on the work of other regulators is to interpret the information they receive and make a decision based on the context of their nation's health care system, their population, and the public health situation in their country. In the approval space, for example, regulators working in countries with intense sunlight and high rates of skin cancers (such as Australia and New Zealand) might come to different decisions regarding the approval of certain dermatological medicines than those working in more temperate climates. This observation underscores another key message: that in the end, it is a national decision as to whether to approve a medicine.

In the beginning of a recognition or reliance relationship, as trust, confidence, and knowledge are being established between two regulatory bodies, it may be said that regulators must "trust but verify." As the relationship strengthens and greater trust is built, the regulators may perceive less of a need to verify each other's work. This decreased need to verify is where regulators can realize further cost savings while remaining confident that public health remains protected. This is critical because in the end, if something goes wrong, it is the responsibility of regulators to explain the decisions they made regarding the status of a product in their market.

Drug Shortages

Drug shortages are a major public health concern for high-, medium-, and low-income countries alike (Iyengar et al., 2016). As a result, patients risk being un- or undertreated for acute or chronic diseases, and the lack of available medicines creates opportunities for substandard and falsified medicines to make their way to consumers. These problems are especially acute for those living in low- and middle-income countries, although those living in higher-income nations are not exempt from the risk. Regulatory authorities, such as FDA, EMA, Australia's Therapeutic Goods Administration, and Health Canada, each have defined approaches and have set up task forces that focus on the problem of drug shortages, collecting data and seeking ways to address the problem. Regulatory authorities' strategies for responding to this public health need include expedited inspections and/or reviews of existing manufacturing sites or new sites (FDA, 2019c). Another strategy is the use of reliance mechanisms. In the case of Mexico, for example, unilateral recognition of the medicines approvals of trusted authorities helped alleviate that country's drug shortages (see Chapter 2), and reliance has also been proposed as a mechanism for helping higher-income nations deal with their drug shortage challenges (Vinther, 2016). Additionally, WHO encourages individual authorities, particularly those in low- and middle-income countries, to rely on products registered on its prequalified medicinal products list to address drug shortages in specific high-priority areas (WHO, 2018a).

Public Health Emergencies

Numerous public health emergencies require quick access to medicinal products. These include, but are not limited to, pandemics, natural disasters, military emergencies, disease outbreaks, and emerging diseases. As is the case with the drug shortages discussed above, government agencies must act in such circumstances to protect the health of their population, and regulatory authorities must weigh the benefits and risks of relaxing more stringent policies and practices.

The Pandemic and All-Hazards Preparedness Reauthorization Act of 2013 empowers FDA to relax regulations so as to expedite access to "medical countermeasures" (e.g., antivirals, antidotes, vaccines, blood products, biological therapeutics) (FDA, 2017a). During public health emergencies, FDA can waive current GMP requirements and make available products it anticipates will be approved in the future, or approve existing drugs for alternative use (FDA, 2017a).

In 2017, Hurricane Maria created an example of a complex public health emergency. The water and debris created a breeding ground for bacteria. Puerto Rican residents were in desperate need of medicines, as they had been injured and exposed to disease-causing bacteria and toxins. Access to already prescribed medicines was hindered by the physical destruction of homes and businesses. In addition to being a public health emergency, the hurricane created shortages of medicines (FDA, 2018d), as 8 percent of all American drug expenditures are on products manufactured in Puerto Rico (FDA, 2017b). In such situations, if regulatory authorities are able to share information via MRAs or other reliance arrangements, they can review assessments of alternative manufacturing sites producing the pharmaceutical products they need.

In a global example, in 2016 WHO declared the Zika virus a public health emergency of international concern (WHO, 2016d). There were no approved tests, vaccines, or treatments for Zika. Researchers and health officials were in constant communication with each other about how to address the problem (WHO, 2016c). As of this writing, Zika was no longer a WHO public health emergency; however, WHO has been encouraging reliance as a way to expedite market access to medicines used to treat and/or prevent priority diseases, given that traditional and/or duplicative inspections by each authority in need of pandemic treatments would result in loss of life (WHO, 2017b).

IMPEDIMENTS TO REGULATORY AUTHORITY RELIANCE

There are numerous impediments to the sharing of information between regulators. Examples of such impediments vary, and might include unusable overly redacted inspection and assessment reports, lack of common formats or standards or conformity, insufficient human and financial resources, conflicts of interest, and insufficient authority granted to regulators entering into informal and formal recognition or reliance arrangements. For regulatory authorities to build further upon their current recognition and reliance activities, impediments to entering into and using informal and formal recognition and reliance arrangements need to be removed. Some impediments originate from within the regulatory authority itself, while others are external to the agency and are influenced by policy makers, industry, or consumer/patient advocacy groups. Each of these stakeholder groups has a role to play in supporting efforts to enhance cooperation with, between, and among regulatory authorities with the aim of improving public health.

Impediments Between Regulatory Authorities

The premise behind sharing a report among regulatory authorities is that an industry sponsor has business interests in all the jurisdictions involved. Reports should be shared only with regulatory authorities representing jurisdictions in which a medicine is being considered for research or market placement. This being the case, it is essential for a regulatory authority with information about a medicine to share that information with a partner regulatory agency identified by an industry sponsor as representing a targeted market. It is equally essential that an industry partner expressing a legitimate intent to conduct business in a jurisdiction also express unambiguous support for that jurisdiction's regulatory authority's gaining full access to assessment reports from partner regulatory authorities. As of this writing, heavily redacted reports represent a significant barrier to the optimal implementation of recognition and reliance arrangements. Unredacted reports (i.e., full reports without parts having been expunged, with the exception of personal privacy information) shared with receiving authorities could be used to inform their decision making. Doing so would uphold the personal privacy protection laws in most jurisdictions and maintain and protect the social contract made with clinical trial participants while facilitating information sharing and optimal execution of recognition and reliance arrangements.

Impediments Between Regulatory Authorities and Industry

The suggestion to ease current redaction practices may contravene current interpretations of trade secret and confidentiality laws in some jurisdictions. However, these laws and precedents were established at a time when most manufacturing was local and were intended to protect a company's legitimate marketing rights in that original jurisdiction, where the regulator had full information as required by law. As discussed in Chapter 1, the current reality is that medicines are no longer primarily local products, but rather global commodities with development, manufacturing, and distribution in many countries; consequently, an examination is needed of whether current trade secret and confidentiality laws, as they apply to information shared between impacted regulatory authorities, are still fit-for-purpose.

Perceived Threats to Sovereignty

It must be emphasized that an agency relying on other countries' work products is neither "outsourcing" that agency's decision making nor giving up sovereignty, accountability, or responsibilities. Agencies retain the ability to make, and the responsibility for making, their own sovereign regulatory decisions. Reliance on materials received through informal information-sharing mechanisms and formal MRAs is, rather, a matter of establishing confidence in the other agency's processes and trust in the information one receives. Such trust usually involves both agencies having a shared public health interest that is fundamental to their decision making. In addition, part of establishing trust is the development of systems for evaluating and validating the quality of the work of other agencies so that when one agency relies on the work of another, it can explain clearly to government officials and its people how it developed the confidence in the other agency that enabled partial or total reliance on information from that agency. Agencies must have the technical capacity, based in robust science and public health, to conduct independent assessments and produce the reports that are shared. With such an arrangement comes the ability to make informed regulatory decisions without having to repeat the assessments of the trusted party. Clearly, avoiding the generation of redundant data for regulatory decision making is one of the main foci of these reliance arrangements. Thus, the receiving regulatory authority exercises sovereignty, interpreting information provided by other regulatory authorities in conjunction with its own information and within the context of the local health care system and public health state of play.

Limited Resources

There are significant costs to developing, adopting, implementing, and maintaining MRAs, particularly in terms of time and human resources (Correia de Brito et al., 2016). For countries establishing GMP MRAs with the EU, trust and confidence in all of the EU Member States must be established. In the case of the EU-US MRA, the agreement mandates that additional resources be used for auditing each EU Member State authority every 5 to 6 years because the actual inspection activities are performed by the individual Member State inspectorates rather than by a central agency inspectorate as in the United States.[4] Often these maintenance costs are not anticipated when the parties first agree to establish an MRA.

Given the increasingly complex therapeutic innovations being tested and brought to market and the growing complexity of medicines supply chains, regulatory authorities will have to consider how relying on others could better ensure the adequate supply of safe and efficacious medicines—the mission of every regulatory authority being to help ensure that patients have access to quality medicines in a well-functioning health care system. In the end, the future of medicines regulation will be found in functional regulatory networks of agencies with increasing specialization and reliance on each other's work, in parallel with decreasing duplicative efforts.

CHALLENGES TO RELIANCE BETWEEN REGULATORY AUTHORITIES IN A GLOBALIZED WORLD

Medicines Production in and Exportation from China and India

Active Pharmaceutical Ingredients

WHO (2017a) has recognized China as an emerging leader in the supply of active pharmaceutical ingredients (APIs). Over the past 30 years,

[4]United States-European Union Amended Sectoral Annex for Pharmaceutical Good Manufacturing Practices (GMP) Appendix 4, Section 3.

China has seen growth in its pharmaceutical manufacturing with respect to the number of facilities and types of manufacturing, and, until recently, without a commensurate development of its medicines regulatory framework (WHO, 2017a). China is now the leading producer and exporter of APIs by volume, manufacturing more than 2,000 APIs (WHO, 2017a). While efforts are under way through cooperative agreements and other regulatory strengthening activities (WHO, 2017a) to help China implement international GMP, it appears that the manufacturing of falsified or substandard medicines and fraudulent clinical and manufacturing data remain challenges in many less resourced manufacturing sites (EMA, 2019d; Rees, 2019a; UNODC, 2019). The international regulatory capacity-building activities being undertaken are helping China better ensure the production of APIs that consistently meet international quality standards. However, the recent drug recall of valsartan highlights the continuing risks associated with the importation of medicines and APIs from countries with less stringent and less consistent regulatory controls (Byrd et al., 2019; EMA, 2019c; WHO, 2017a).

Generics

India, like China, is a major supplier of generic medicines to the world. According to the India Brand Equity Foundation (IBEF, 2019), the Indian pharmaceutical sector accounts for 71 percent of the market share of generic drugs and supplies more than 50 percent of the world's vaccines. While the generics industry remains robust in India, the government has signaled a desire to expand its market while also making India a major hub for low-cost drug research and development (Indian Department of Pharmaceuticals, 2018). Yet, FDA and other regulators document repeated problems with quality manufacturing at many of the Indian sites that wish to export products to their countries (Rees, 2019b).

A Changing World

China has aspirations to shift the primary focus of its manufacturing from APIs for export to the more lucrative export of finished products and to become a world leader in research and development. However, it does not appear this will happen in the immediate future (Ni et al., 2017; WHO, 2017a). India, Brazil, and other middle-income countries also have aspirations to increase their abilities to develop and produce new medicines for both local and global consumption. These aspirations for expanding markets speak to the larger issue that the pharmaceutical landscape is constantly evolving and changing. India and China may be the world's major suppliers of APIs and generics in today's market, but as production costs in

China and India rise, new countries may enter into those market segments. Regulators need to be prepared for such shifts in the landscape to ensure the quality, safety, and efficacy of medicines regardless of the location of their production.

In addition, the pharmaceutical industry is continually advancing. The entire drug research and development enterprise is globalizing rapidly. Regulators cannot remain static in their acquisition of knowledge and their incorporation of the talent needed to understand new technological advances in precision medicine and drug development. It will be impossible to predict the exact skills needed to ensure the quality, safety, and efficacy of complex and innovative medicinal products such as complex biologics and gene and cell therapies. However, the establishment of a strong system of reliance can build a network of trusted experts from different agencies that can be drawn upon for their valuable insight when a product development or assessment challenge arises that has not previously been encountered or addressed.

The Need for Mutual Recognition of Third-Country Inspections

Given the large number of manufacturing sites in China and India that are involved in producing drug components and/or final products for the United States and Europe, it has not been possible for either FDA or EMA to inspect all of these sites as they would like to do in order to assure the quality of products being exported to their people. However, recent updates to the EU-US MRA on pharmaceutical GMP do make provisions for mutual recognition of inspections conducted by the parties to the MRA in third countries.[5] Although these provisions regarding recognition of third-country inspections have not yet been implemented, the expectation is that this MRA, which became operational in July 2019, will allow greater sharing between regulatory bodies in the United States and Europe. This increased sharing will avoid duplication of efforts, thereby allowing those

[5]Art. 1 "The provisions of this Annex apply to pharmaceutical inspections of manufacturing facilities carried out in the territory of a Party during the marketing of products (hereafter referred to as 'post-approval inspections') and, to the extent provided for in Article 11, before products are marketed (hereafter referred to as 'pre-approval inspections'), **as well as, to the extent provided for in Article 8.3, to pharmaceutical inspections of manufacturing facilities carried out outside the territory of either Party.**" [emphasis added]

Art. 8.3 "**A Party may accept official GMPs documents issued by a recognized authority of the other Party for manufacturing facilities located outside the territory of the issuing authority.**" [emphasis added] (Brussels, 1.3.2017 C(2017) 1323 final ANNEX to the Commission Decision on determining the Union position for a Decision of the Joint Committee set up under Article 14 of the Agreement on Mutual Recognition between the European Community and the United States of America, in order to amend the Sectoral Annex on Pharmaceutical Good Manufacturing Practices [GMPs].)

regulators to redistribute their inspectional resources to higher-risk facilities both within their own borders and in third countries.

Predating the 2019 implementation of the EU-US MRA was the International API Inspection Program, which had grown from a pilot to a full program by 2011. The program created a framework for greater international collaboration and information sharing on GMP inspections of API manufacturers worldwide (EMA, 2018a). In 2016, it included regulatory agencies from Australia, Canada, Denmark, France, Germany, Ireland, Italy, Japan, the United Kingdom, and the United States.[6] The work focused primarily on sharing plans for, outcomes of, and reports stemming from the GMP inspections. Most of the information shared was through monthly teleconferences and electronic exchanges. A spreadsheet (the Master List) of all API sites of interest to all those participating in the program formed the foundation for a mapping exercise carried out by the International Coalition of Medicines Regulatory Authorities showing the API manufacturing sites of common interest. This information is currently stored in the secure European database for GMP and good distribution practice inspections and certification platform, EudraGMDP, where participating countries take responsibility for updating their own information. Box 3-2 provides a summary of an evaluation of the program, and Appendix C presents a chart, adapted from the work of the International Coalition of Medicines Regulatory Authorities, showing the objective, scope, membership, and work products of global initiatives (EMA, 2016).

[6]The European Directorate for the Quality of Medicines and HealthCare from the Council of Europe and WHO were also considered members; Germany's engagement ended in 2016.

BOX 3-2
Summary of the International API Inspection Program Evaluation

An evaluation of the International API Inspection Program, which helped lay a foundation for collaboration among medicines regulators, was conducted between 2011 and 2016. Analysis of the results revealed the number of sites of common interest to regulatory authorities (see the table below). This common interest is particularly notable between the U.S. Food and Drug Administration (FDA) and participating European authorities, with 350 sites of common interest. Also of note are the 944 recorded good manufacturing practice (GMP) inspections conducted over the 6 years at 458 sites (49 percent in India and 36 percent in China), and the number of duplicate inspections at sites that were in compliance with GMP standards, which totaled 358. The authors of the evaluation report do not state where the duplications occurred, but they do comment on continued efforts aimed at reducing the number of duplicate inspections. The authors further assert that through increased cooperation and information sharing, duplication of effort was diminished, and human resources were channeled to unique sites, increasing overall inspection coverage.

Number of Sites of Common Interest Shared Between at Least Two Participating Authorities

	TGA	FDA	WHO
European authorities*	136	350	41
TGA	x	176	17
FDA	x	x	50

NOTES: FDA = U.S. Food and Drug Administration; TGA = Australian Therapeutic Goods Administration; WHO = World Health Organization.
*Including the European Directorate for the Quality of Medicines and HealthCare.
SOURCE: EMA, 2018a.

4

Stakeholder Views of Recognition and Reliance

This chapter draws heavily on information-gathering sessions conducted by the committee between April and August 2019. In these sessions, current and former regulators and representatives of international harmonization initiatives, industry, and patient advocacy groups gave presentations and answered questions from the committee. These speakers brought numerous challenges, benefits, and opportunities associated with recognition and reliance arrangements to light. Appendix D includes the agendas for the public where key stakeholders informed the work of this committee by providing views and perspectives that were considered in preparing this report. To the extent possible, points raised by stakeholders about issues related to regulatory challenges and opportunities entailed in recognition and reliance arrangements were compiled into listings presented in this chapter. Content for these listings was supplemented by stakeholder written responses to committee questions, a questionnaire administered by the World Health Organization (WHO), the published literature, and publicly available government reports. The final section of the chapter presents the committee's synthesis of the challenges and opportunities thus derived.

VIEWS OF STAKEHOLDERS

To simply say "the world is changing rapidly" hardly captures the conditions under which medicines regulators are currently working. This was a subtle message expressed by stakeholders throughout all of the committee's information-gathering work. As of this writing, there was uncertainty about the future of the United Kingdom as part of the European Union (EU) and what that would mean for the Medicines & Healthcare products Regulatory Agency and its colleagues within the European Network. There was also more offshore manufacturing of drugs taking place than ever before. Such a shift requires that more regulators spend time in those countries where the manufacturing is taking place—in 2019, that was China and India (see Chapter 3). This was not the case just two decades earlier, and whether these two countries will remain the dominant producers of generics a decade from now is yet another uncertainty.

Just as the global landscape is changing, so too are medicines regulatory bodies' recognition and reliance arrangements, the staff that design them, and the parties involved. Therefore, it must be emphasized that what is presented in this chapter represents a snapshot in time. The committee recognizes that circumstances may have changed even by the time this report is published. In an effort to present relevant material in a constantly changing environment, this chapter is organized around themes intended to help guide the discussion of a core set of challenges and opportunities associated with reliance arrangements in the following chapter.

Impediments and Challenges

Presented in Box 4-1 is a list of impediments that could stall or inhibit communication and collaboration among medicines regulators, thereby preventing any type of meaningful recognition or reliance. This is followed by more targeted messages captured in Box 4-2 about challenges specific to reliance in conducting good manufacturing practice (GMP) inspections, as well as more general challenges that could be faced with any type of reliance used within medicines regulation.

Benefits and Opportunities

The potential contribution of improved decision making to protecting the public health was a clear message from the regulators who provided input for this study, as was the potential to facilitate focusing limited resources on higher-risk issues. It is critically important to understand these points given that ensuring safe and efficacious quality medicines for the health of society is key to the mission of medicines regulatory authorities. For example, greater information sharing between national regulators and national health systems in the form of early-stage notification could help limit the effects of a public health event caused by a medicine. Currently, the Pharmaceutical Inspection Co-operation Scheme (PIC/S) has a procedure for alerting other authorities about recalls arising from quality defects in medicinal products (PIC/S, 2017), and WHO has a system for notifying authorities about products found to be substandard or falsified. The system

BOX 4-1
Impediments to International Communication and Collaboration

- Resource constraints, staff turnover, and shifting agency priorities present risks to maximizing information sharing.
- The maximal benefits of information sharing between trusted regulatory authorities will not be realized without the full engagement of participating regulatory authorities and the ability to share full, unredacted reports.
- Lack of a shared database with a comprehensive list of registered, uniquely identified active pharmaceutical ingredient manufacturers leads to an inability to anticipate future inspections and therefore to develop a plan for avoiding duplicate inspections.
- Lack of a common policy framework for the inspection of shared sites located in third countries limits the ability of regulatory authorities to use other authorities' inspection reports or to reduce the number of duplicative inspections.
- Lack of transparency and visibility of inspection reports that can be shared with and used by lower-resourced regulatory authorities limits reliance capability.

SOURCES: Information-gathering sessions; EMA, 2018a.

BOX 4-2
Challenges Within Regulatory Reliance

Challenges with Reliance on Good Manufacturing Practice Inspections Among Well-Resourced Regulatory Authorities

- Lack of transparency—particular challenge of redacted assessment reports for obtaining information needed to make an informed regulatory decision
- Lack of expertise—for highly innovative products, absence of the same level of expertise everywhere now and in the future
- Existing differences in regulatory systems
- Investment costs—need for up-front and sustained investments of resources to realize benefits:
  - Potential that benefits may not be realized until much later because of the time and resources needed to develop trust, increase knowledge, and achieve convergence
  - Need to foster an understanding that reliance is not an opportunity to reduce resources used by participating regulatory authorities, but rather an assurance that agencies can avoid duplication and focus their resources on key activities that bring value to the populations they serve (i.e., more efficient use of resources in areas of higher public health risk in which they cannot rely on others)
- Lack of secure information technology systems—lack of secure platforms and procedures for the exchange and management of nonpublic information

continued

BOX 4-2 Continued

- Mindset—perception among regulators that reliance reduces autonomy or the belief that reliance is "outsourcing" one's regulatory responsibilities or accountabilities
- Resource misfits—possibility that the decrease in inspections as a result of mutual recognition agreements and other forms of reliance may not translate to an increase in inspections at other sites because of legal restrictions or skillset deficiencies that hinder the movement of inspectors from one site to another
  - For example, inability to transfer inspectors with expertise in assessing biotechnology companies to active pharmaceutical ingredient manufacturing sites because the required expertise is different
  - Similarly, the possibility that staff with expertise in one specialty area may not be motivated to conduct inspections in another
- Differing assessment methods—possibility that benefit/risk assessments of drugs differ for different partners
- Coordinating schedules for collaborative activities

Challenges for Any Form of Reliance

- Insufficient resources given increasing globalization and global complexities
- Differences in regulatory systems
- Time required to build trust and confidence
- Need for buy-in from key stakeholders, including industry
- Need for buy-in from agency reviewers and inspectors who may fear that reliance reduces autonomy, stringency, and job security
- Lack of an assessment strategy and metrics for measuring and documenting the success of an agreement or arrangement
- Difficulty in objectively measuring outcomes of reliance arrangements
- Political challenges outside of medicines regulation

SOURCES: Cooke, 2019; WHO, 2016a,b.

also includes a rapid notification procedure for alerting regulatory authorities of counterfeit or tampered products when urgent action is required to protect public health. The system is dependent on the submission of this information by regulators. According to the regulators who provided input for this study, the system works fairly well, although there is room for improvement. Currently, this system is dependent primarily on external resources, and staffing is limited relative to the system's mandate.

Benefits of Reliance

Boxes 4-3 and 4-4 list a number of benefits expressed by respondents regarding reliance in areas other than GMP—medicines approval decisions

BOX 4-3
Benefits and Perceived Benefits of Reliance in Medicines Approval Decisions

- Regulatory functions are more efficient, with faster review and shorter times to approval.
  - Faster market availability can improve global public health.
  - Faster access to medicines is particularly valuable for countries with smaller medicines markets, which generally receive marketing applications later than countries/regions with larger markets.
- Sharing of information relating to noncompliance with good clinical practice facilitates the prioritization of internal resources.
- For countries that do not conduct inspections abroad, sharing of inspection certificates by partner nations is very valuable to their risk-based regulatory decision-making process.

BOX 4-4
Benefits of International Communication and Collaboration

- Information can be shared.
- Trust can be built that elevates confidence in participants.
- Transparency and visibility of inspection reports can promote global public health by facilitating better utilization of global inspection resources to focus on higher-risk facilities.
- Inspections of previously inspected sites can be deferred.
- Regularly scheduled teleconferences can allow for clarifying conversations and more detailed discussions about information shared in inspection reports.
- Shared inspection reports can stimulate a desire for joint inspections.
- Metrics can be used to determine elements of programs with the highest return on investment.

and international communication and collaboration, respectively. Because so much of the discussion with stakeholders involved mutual recognition agreements (MRAs) and thus GMP, Box 4-5 lists separately the perceived and real benefits of reliance in the area of GMP based on the sources described previously. It must be emphasized that "perceived" does not mean the benefits are not real, without ex post evaluations; however, it is impossible to know whether the benefits describing greater regulatory efficiency, for example, have actually been attained. Nonetheless, for this particular example, there are indications of expected cost savings from the

BOX 4-5
Perceived Benefits of Reliance in Good Manufacturing Practice (GMP) Inspections

- Increased knowledge and trust between and among regulatory partners
  - More informed decision making
  - Joint inspections or observed inspections between mutual recognition agreement (MRA) partners that further increase knowledge of and trust in the other partners
  - Cooperation and collaboration that increase mutual confidence among GMP inspections field regulators
  - Sharing of unredacted reports that promotes confidence and trust
- Regulatory efficiency (faster review and time to approval)
  - Early distribution of information on sites identified as GMP noncompliant facilitated
  - Ability to react quickly in case of rapid alerts
- More effective use of resources
  - Better use of resources through better communication, coordination, and collaboration on sites of common interest
  - Inspection prioritization and risk-based inspection planning facilitated
  - Duplication of effort reduced
  - Resources directed toward manufacturers posing higher risks
- Improved quality of reviews/inspections/overall regulatory system
  - Continuous improvement process for all partners supported by regular, joint audits
- Improved global public health
  - Reallocation of resources that allows for more inspections in third countries of active pharmaceutical ingredient and finished-product manufacturers, ensuring that higher-risk and more total manufacturing sites are inspected
  - Regularly scheduled discussions on medicine shortages and genetically modified domestic products
  - Scientific and procedural deliberation, promoted by the process of achieving recognition and reliance, which likely leads to more informed decision making and increased patient safety
  - Inspection of various sites and various product categories using global resources/expertise facilitated by information sharing
  - Companies' greater willingness to enter countries with smaller markets and lower purchasing power/return on industry investment
- Increased empowerment for smaller regulatory bodies
  - Stronger voice for smaller authorities due to reliance collaborations, which may drive convergence and influence developments and guidelines in areas that may be beneficial to these smaller national medicines regulatory authorities
  - Ability of small market/small regulatory bodies to maximize their limited resources for achieving the best outcomes while retaining a high degree of regulatory stringency and sovereign decision making

recently activated US-EU MRA. The European Commission estimates that 100 inspections in the United States will be waived by the end of 2019. One inspection takes roughly 16 person-days for the regulatory authority and 160 person-days for industry (at an estimated cost for industry of €352,000 or $389,493) (EFPIA, 2018). The benefits listed in Box 4-5 include those associated with a regulatory authority's relying, to some extent, on other regulatory agencies for GMP inspection information instead of performing such inspections itself.

Opportunities for Reliance

Whereas benefits represent gains stakeholders perceive as having accrued to them through reliance arrangements, opportunities represent gains they hope to realize through greater reliance in regulatory environments. Box 4-6 lists opportunities identified by stakeholders, both those related specifically to reliance within GMP and those that might go beyond GMP. Discussions of good laboratory practice (GLP) and good clinical practice (GCP) during the committee's information-gathering sessions were more limited than those of GMP; however, they yielded some outlook that the expansion of the EU-US MRA into areas beyond GMP and batch certification would require political will. Reliance for market authorization—the approval process for medicinal products—would entail sharing of robust data that could be analyzed extensively and completely so that all parties would understand the conclusions reached, which could be difficult for complex medicinal products. However, the situation is different for variations in marketing authorizations of medicines. In this case, the source product is already on the market, so that verification of the risks and benefits for its use in patients already exist. The EU system does accept "do-and-tell" whereby companies make some changes after a product is on the market and then inform the regulators. Because this process does not require an assessment, companies are expected to make the necessary changes, and these reports could easily be shared. The situation is different for companies seeking changes in medicines that could modify their risk/benefit profile (e.g., a new indication, a change in dosing, or the addition of new elements in the safety profile). Because this situation requires an assessment, sharing in this space would require political will. Therefore, one way forward would be to start small and evolve toward this outcome.

The committee's focus on GMP does not indicate less importance for GLP or GCP, just relatively less input from stakeholders. This limited input may reflect time restrictions for the committee's interviews, or a potential gap in the shared work of regulators and a potential opportunity for future reliance arrangements. For example, given that most drug development employs multiregional clinical trials to provide the clinical evidence for

BOX 4-6
Opportunities Within Reliance for Good Manufacturing Practice (GMP) Inspections, as Well as Other Areas

Opportunities in GMP

- Increased transparency—broadening discussions regarding how reference agencies provide assessment or inspection outcomes (e.g., with respect to redactions, online options, timing efficiency)
  - Sharing unredacted reports could promote an understanding of reviewed material and the rationale for decisions made
  - Sharing unredacted reports could promote confidence and trust
  - Relying on a redacted document is usually not possible and often leads to the need to conduct what is a redundant activity to obtain the redacted information
- Harmonized forms—including more discrete data fields or structured-format content to better leverage foreign inspections
- Better use of information technology—providing assessment or inspection outcomes (GMP certificates or inspection reports)
- Aligned interests—expanding the scope of an already-planned inspection to include other authorities' areas of interest
- Communication and capacity building—building on work done by international organizations such as the International Coalition of Medicines Regulatory Authorities and the Pharmaceutical Inspection Co-operation Scheme (PIC/S) to enhance communication and information sharing on GMP-related inspections
  - Experiences, plans, and best practices could be discussed among medicines regulators at international workshops on reliance
  - Capacity and trust building between regulators could be encouraged through international efforts (e.g., by sharing information on and mutual participation in training activities)

marketing authorization, such trials are fairly common for both the United States and the EU (EMA, 2009a); therefore, citizens from both jurisdictions may be participants in the same global clinical trial. Both U.S. and EU regulators are required to verify that any study under their jurisdiction—whether in-country or abroad—has followed GCP, was conducted in an ethical manner, and reported accurate and complete data. Given globalization and resource limitations, inspection of all clinical trial sites is virtually impossible. One answer to this challenge is to create greater efficiencies through collaboration in GCP inspections and the exchange of information and inspection reports. Indeed, the European Medicines Agency and the U.S. Food and Drug Administration tested this possibility under their arrangement. The pilot test ended in 2011 and could provide the founda-

- Efforts under way to converge/harmonize inspection processes and reports could be maximized within PIC/S
- Human resource development—identifying the most appropriate experts from an international pool of specialists to conduct inspections aligned with their expertise and/or capacity
- Evaluation—establishing and/or sharing metrics for evaluating reliance arrangements
  - Uptake of reliance pathways could be a useful impact measure for reliance efforts

Opportunities in Other Areas

- Proactive sharing of post-market safety data
- Establishment of standards for timeliness and minimum information content for posting emergent safety issues or regulatory actions
- Standardization of good pharmacovigilance practices, including roles and responsibilities of industry in collecting foreign safety data
- Reliance/work sharing in the area of pharmacovigilance, post-authorization safety, and efficacy monitoring
- Access to additional expertise on post-market actions, facilitating responses to issues
- Full access to the European Union (EU) database (EudraGMDP) and thus full access to noncompliance statements, manufacturing licenses, and GMP certificates granted for all EU mutual recognition agreement (MRA) partners
- U.S. Food and Drug Administration (FDA) database for information sharing under the EU-US MRA
- Verification of GMP compliance of U.S. sites allowed for by Market Authorisation Application

SOURCES: Cooke, 2019; WHO, 2016b.

tion for future expansion of the recently activated EU-US MRA. Other regulators might also consider exploring the feasibility of reliance in this area.

A Patient-Centered Regulatory Framework

Virtually all of the regulators who provided input for this study supported the notion that each reliance arrangement either does now or would in the future enable medicines regulatory agencies to improve their efficiency. The regulators also agreed that such arrangements allow them to redirect resources to areas of greater need, although none had data from their agency to support that claim. However, that lack of data may change with the EU-US MRA, as the partners agreed to establish performance indicators with which to demonstrate that implementing the agreement would deliver what had been promised. Information on the specific metrics were not shared with the committee, although a patient advocate from the International Alliance of Patients' Organizations expressed his interest in what might be measured through the development of a framework that put the patient or consumer at its core. He stressed that in such a framework, patient safety would have to be paramount. He also highlighted the importance of ensuring faster access to innovations, particularly gene therapies and biotherapeutics, through MRAs or other reliance arrangements, so that patients who needed these innovative medicines would have access to them. Furthermore, he stressed the need for measuring increased equity, especially in the area of rare diseases, where patients stand to benefit most from increased reliance and access to new medicines. Lastly, his patient-centered framework would include metrics for affordability. He encouraged policy makers to invite patients into debates about regulatory reliance in general and MRAs in particular, emphasizing that patients can offer a real-life perspective that is often missing from policy-driven conversations. He also believes patients could bring a unique view to GMP inspections.

Industry Perspective

The pharmaceutical industry has benefited from recognition and reliance arrangements, as the collaboration that takes place provides guidelines for industry. In other words, it becomes clearer to all parties what is needed to facilitate market authorization across multiple jurisdictions. There are many agreed-upon technical requirements; however, when a consensus is lacking as to all of the information to be relied on, the approval process decelerates. Applications for different regulatory authorities have different requirements and these inconsistencies diminish their ability to rely on each other's work products. Moreover, as medicines continue to become more complex, the burden of duplicative inspections on industry will increase, and the benefit to multiple jurisdictions will be small, as the expertise necessary to examine complex medicines effectively may be limited to a few individuals.

Acknowledging the complications associated with initiating and implementing MRAs, industry still sees opportunities for MRAs to expand reliance beyond GMP. Attention focuses on product review and first approval inspections; however, a large percentage of industry work occurs in the post-approval and lifecycle management spaces, which are as important to public health as initial approvals. Regulatory authorities have limited capacity, resulting in backlog such that several years may pass before they are able to review post-approval changes, hindering multinational distribution. Regulatory reliance has potential utility across the medicines lifecycle; examples include registration, inspections, variations, post-approval changes, import testing, and lot release. For example, MRAs and other reliance arrangements used for post-approval changes to vaccine supply would motivate industry because expedited market penetration would be secured. The opportunity to reduce the time and effort put forth to keep essential medicines on the market parallels regulatory authorities' goal of reducing supply shortages.

SYNTHESIZING THE CHALLENGES AND OPPORTUNITIES

Understanding the Value of Reliance

Of particular note from the committee-developed supplemental information-gathering questionnaire and information-gathering sessions was the importance of helping all stakeholders understand that increased reliance is not an opportunity simply to reduce the resource needs or fees of participating regulatory authorities. Rather, reliance presents opportunities for ensuring that agencies can avoid duplication and focus their resources on key activities that bring value to the populations they serve instead of repeating redundant regulatory tasks. If full trust is built, the result may be greater public health protection. Currently, the overwhelming perception of all the stakeholders whose views were gathered for this study is that greater recognition and reliance in all their forms will, in both the short and long terms, strengthen public health across the globe.

Financial Implications

Among the challenges associated with reliance arrangements, particularly in the case of MRAs, are the costs of setting them up. In most cases, these costs are short term, as they are related to the high degree of administrative and programmatic effort needed to develop, negotiate, and maintain the arrangement. The financial benefits are believed to be realized once the arrangement has been fully implemented. Expected gains in financial and time efficiencies may be modest in the initial phases of trust and knowledge building, but what must be emphasized is the improved decision-making process that is realized when two or more sets of national regulators work together. The stakeholders interviewed by the committee reported their view that this benefit more than compensates for the initial investment of time and resources (see the opportunities listed in Box 4-6). In addition to regulators, these arrangements provide benefits to both industry and consumers. Industry stands to benefit through improved market access, fewer duplicative inspections, and batch retesting waivers upon importation, each of which could translate into greater financial return for companies and indirectly generate public health benefits (e.g., a reduction in redundant regulatory processes expedites the availability of products to populations in need). For patients and consumers, reliance arrangements can provide access to a wider array of medicines at potentially lower cost, as was expressed by the speaker discussing the work of Mexico's Comisión Federal para la Protección contra Riesgos Sanitarios in recognizing generic approvals of trusted authorities (see Chapter 2). The overall outcome of these benefits is improved public health protection.

Transparency

As was discussed with stakeholders, a potentially more sustainable model than unilateral reliance might involve greater transparency of the work of well- and moderately well-resourced regulatory bodies that are performing at an international level of regulatory oversight. Increased information sharing along with efforts—such as those of WHO and PIC/S—at capability and capacity building among lower-resourced regulatory authorities could improve overall global public health while opening the door to better-informed sovereign decision making in all countries, regardless of national income status. The availability of unredacted reports would allow both well- and lower-resourced regulatory authorities to perform their regulatory activities in an ever-improving manner. One of the issues for lower-resourced regulators is that the medicines involved may be different, so it is important for them to understand the details provided in a shared report. In some cases, it is not possible to truly rely on the work product of another agency unless the receiving agency obtains a full report. The availability of such unredacted reports would both allow other countries to use these reports to reach their own sovereign decisions on market access and help build needed capabilities in review capacity among regulatory authorities.

Public Health Imperative

The public health imperative drives some countries to expand their participation in reliance arrangements. In the case of New Zealand, for example, the population is relatively small and thus may be a lower marketing priority for multinational drug companies compared with larger markets. An MRA with Australia, however, has enabled the New Zealand authority to incentivize sponsors to submit for marketing authorization in that country. This mechanism will contribute to bringing new drugs to New Zealand in a timely manner despite the country's limited market size and population. It should be noted that many countries ensure access to innovative medicines without mutual arrangements—they just unilaterally recognize marketing authorizations issued by other regulatory authorities with the capacity to assess such products. Without such unilateral arrangements, new medicines would not reach many countries in the world. It is speculated that such a process, if built on a foundation of trust, might even be a faster mechanism for approving medicines and getting them to these markets relative to using an MRA.

As discussed previously, informal arrangements that facilitate decision making through reliance on the exchange of trusted information include Memoranda of Understanding, confidentiality commitments, regularly scheduled discussions, and agreed-upon work-sharing programs. In these situations, agencies are gaining access to trusted information that they can then use to decide whether further action on their part is needed prior to making a regulatory decision, or they can make their sovereign regulatory decision informed, in part or in whole, by the information received through these informal arrangements.

5

Removing Impediments and Facilitating Action for Greater Recognition and Reliance Among Regulatory Authorities

Based on its extensive deliberations and input from stakeholders representing regulatory authorities, international organizations, industry, and patient groups, the committee identified key challenges and opportunities that led it to draw one conclusion and offer six recommendations. In the course of its discussions and online searches, the committee also came to realize that stakeholder groups other than regulators have an interest in seeing regulatory authorities overcome impediments to greater regulatory cooperation. Because of their motivation, the committee has incorporated each of these groups—industry representatives, patient advocates, policy makers, and regulators themselves—into a proposed strategy in which each has responsibility for helping all regulators across the spectrum of country resources overcome impediments to achieving effective recognition and reliance.

This strategy, along with the committee's conclusion and recommendations, stems from two overarching messages that serve as the lens through which the committee's conclusion and recommendations should be viewed:

- Regulation through recognition and reliance arrangements is now a 21st-century best regulatory practice. Accordingly, regulators, regardless of human, technical, and financial resources, should make increased use of reliance and cooperation with other trusted regulators, as no regulator has the resources it needs to meet all of its public health responsibilities.
- Impediments to regulators entering into and using such informal and formal recognition and reliance arrangements to help them

obtain the information they need for their regulatory decision making should be removed.

It is safe to say that virtually all regulatory authorities are motivated by a public health mission to safeguard their populations with respect to the medicines coming into and currently on the market in their jurisdictions. Additionally, given the rapid movement of people and illnesses across borders in today's world, it is similarly safe to say that public health is a global concern and that all regulators, regardless of size or financial resources, exercise their responsibilities within that global public health framework as part of a larger global regulatory enterprise. How regulatory authorities carry out their missions and structure their regulatory cooperation activities is often a function of human and financial resources.

MEDICINES REGULATION IN A GLOBALIZED WORLD

Challenge

Every year, billions of people around the world take prescription medicines. The pharmaceutical industry has expanded its production in an effort to meet this massive demand for drugs, while producers of generics and biosimilars are attempting to help meet the demand with lower-priced alternatives. The pharmaceutical industry has looked to reduce its expenses by moving production and manufacturing to locations with lower associated costs. An end result has been the mixing of ingredients from different overseas sources. Today, drug manufacturers rely on vast networks of subcontractors for medicine production, sometimes working with as many as 200 contracted manufacturing organizations covering different functions, such as production of active pharmaceutical ingredients (APIs), bulk production, and finished product packaging (Office of the Director of National Intelligence, 2018). Other vendors handle additional aspects of providing power, water, and hazardous waste disposal.

Challenge: Rapid globalization of drug discovery, research and development, manufacturing, and delivery has significant implications for public health. The resources required to ensure comprehensive oversight of these activities is now an overwhelming task for even the well-resourced national medicines regulatory agencies. All have limited resources to accomplish well all the tasks they are asked to perform. The ongoing evolution of the science and technology associated with drug discovery, research and development, manufacturing, and delivery (e.g., dramatic increases in more complex biological medicines and emerging use of cell and gene therapies) poses additional capacity challenges for regulatory agencies. These challenges underline the need for further cooperation and collaboration among agencies; however, achieving that cooperation is often challenging because individual agencies have different histories, legal frameworks, resources, and areas of expertise.

Opportunity

It is the responsibility of industry to monitor its own, globalized supply chains and to correct and report any issues that may arise during manufacturing and production processes. Regulatory agencies are expected to ensure that industry takes the proper steps so that people within their jurisdiction have access to safe and effective quality medicines; good manufacturing practice (GMP) is essential to that assurance. According to Patel and Chotai (2011), GMP diminishes the risk of cross-contamination, labeling errors, and other such inaccuracies that may represent a particular vulnerability given the wide array of international subcontractors with which industry works in deriving a final product.

Just as the manufacture and production of medicines now represent a global undertaking, research and development toward the approval of new medicines has expanded in an attempt to capture more of a global market while minimizing costs associated with drug development. Good laboratory practice (GLP) regulations help ensure that nonclinical studies on product safety are adequately planned and performed and reflect sufficiently documented, trustworthy data (Andrade et al., 2016). In the Organisation for Economic Co-operation and Development (OECD) global context—which extends beyond medicines—GLP principles provide "a common basis for cooperation among national authorities and avoid[s] creating non-tariff barriers to trade" (OECD, 2019).

OECD has issued a document on the governance of clinical trials (OECD, 2013b). In that document, the authors note that approximately 25 percent of clinical trial applications involved two or more OECD member states and that roughly two-thirds of all subjects enrolled in clinical trials were part of multinational studies. Conducting such studies is costly. To reduce expenses, among other purposes, trials are increasingly including non-U.S. and non–Western European participants (Ravinetto et al., 2016). Good clinical practice (GCP) guidelines for ensuring the ethical treatment of study subjects are currently being reviewed in light of the high volume of globalized clinical trials and the challenges this poses for all regulatory authorities reviewing multinational studies.

As was stated in interviews conducted for this study, the closer a regulatory agency's framework is to that of another agency, the more likely it is that collaborative efforts will lead toward recognition and reliance. For example, Health Canada and the Therapeutic Goods Administration of Australia (TGA) have equivalent regulatory frameworks and also overlap in language, paving the way for reliance activities and their mutual recognition agreement (MRA). These two medium-sized regulatory authorities teamed up with two other "like-minded" agencies in Singapore and Switzerland for their successful work-sharing initiative, the Australia-Canada-Singapore-Switzerland Consortium.

In some ways, the U.S. Food and Drug Administration (FDA) stands alone with regard to its high level of resources, but in many other ways, it shares similarities with other moderately well- and well-resourced regulatory authorities. For example, both the European Medicines Agency (EMA) and FDA struggle with challenges posed by advanced therapeutics such as gene therapy, somatic cell therapy, and tissue-engineered products (Hunter, 2017). These and other innovations in medicine are testing the boundaries of countries' regulatory processes as the agencies try to stay ahead of the science for ensuring safety without stifling innovation. Given that FDA and EMA align through their commitment to drug development standards and their adoption of International Council for Harmonisation of Technical Requirements for Pharmaceuticals for Human Use guidelines, these agencies are well positioned to expand on the information sharing and collaboration conducted within their confidentiality arrangement (Kashoki et al., 2020). Cluster activities, initially set up through EMA and FDA, provide regularly scheduled opportunities for sharing on specific topics with other similarly situated authorities. The advanced-therapy medicinal products cluster includes EMA, FDA, and Health Canada. A biosimilars cluster has representatives from these agencies plus Japan's Pharmaceuticals and Medical Devices Agency. This cluster works toward greater alignment of biosimilar evaluations that could allow for increased acceptance of data across regulatory bodies (EMA, 2019e).

Opportunity: In confronting the global challenges of medicines regulation, cooperation and collaboration among regulators offer opportunities to share information and increase the transparency of each other's activities; to share finite resources and address the growing workload resulting from globalization; and to rely on each other's processes, work products, and decision making via both formal reliance arrangements such as MRAs and other, less formal reliance arrangements.

Conclusion: The committee concludes that protecting and promoting public health in a time of globalization and unprecedented advances in technology and medicines—which are mirrored by the growing complexity of medicines and the supply chains for their manufacture and production—is the single greatest challenge facing medicines regulatory authorities today. It is therefore imperative that regulatory authorities at all resource levels—well, moderately well, and lower—find ways to continue or expand on their ability and willingness to work together to maximize the use of their finite resources so they can ensure the quality, safety, efficacy, and availability of medicines for their jurisdiction in both emergency and non-emergency situations.

However, for regulatory authorities to further build on their current recognition and reliance activities, impediments to entering into and using formal and informal recognition and reliance arrangements need to be removed. Some of these impediments are within the regulatory authority itself while others may be external to the agency and influenced by those within policy, industry, or consumer/patient advocacy groups. Each of these stakeholder groups has a role to play in supporting efforts to enhance cooperation between and among regulatory authorities, with the overarching aim of improving public health. The committee therefore recommends that all regulatory authorities and other key stakeholder groups demonstrate their support for formal and informal medicines regulatory recognition and reliance arrangements using a targeted approach.

Recommendation 1: The committee recommends a strategy that leverages the support of each stakeholder group in the following manner:

- **All regulatory authorities, especially those that are well- and moderately well-resourced, should increase information sharing and the transparency of each other's regulatory activities across the lifecycle of medicines in ways that can facilitate more efficient resource allocation and decision making for all regulators and reduce the burden of redundant regulatory activities on regulators, patients, and industry.**
- **All regulatory authorities, especially those that are well- and moderately well-resourced, should be allowed to share their work products in essentially unredacted form (i.e., full reports without parts of the report expunged, except for personal privacy information) with other regulatory authorities so assessment and inspection information can be made available to those other regulators, especially those that are lower-resourced, thereby enabling access to quality, usable regulatory information by a greater number of regulatory authorities for addressing global public health needs. In this respect, policy makers, and the U.S. Congress in particular, should weigh the challenges and opportunities involved in empowering their respective medicines regulatory authorities to share complete, unredacted inspection reports (e.g., good manufacturing practice**

reports) with other regulatory authorities so as to facilitate learning, aid in decision making, reduce the use of limited resources on redundant inspections, decrease the burden on industry of redundant inspections, and strengthen the overall global public heath infrastructure for safe and effective quality medicines.

- **Lower-resourced regulatory authorities should consider the risks and benefits of unilateral recognition of the regulatory decisions of trusted regulatory authorities when doing so would facilitate better public health decision making in the context in which the lower-resourced regulatory authority functions.**
- **Industry should support the recognition and reliance efforts of regulatory authorities by encouraging them to share less redacted or, better, unredacted reports with their trusted regulatory authority partners, and by showing a willingness to share health-related data and/or information relevant to regulatory decision making more publicly to benefit the global public health good and reduce the sharing authority's own burden of redundant oversight.**
- **Patient and consumer groups should support the recognition and reliance efforts of medicines regulatory authorities by advocating for a "public health protection and promotion" framing of all such arrangements and for their increased use.**

The committee further believes, based on its information gathering and expert opinion, that formal and informal recognition and reliance arrangements are very effective tools for facilitating cooperation and reliance on the work of other regulatory authorities when they are established in ways that emphasize public health, maximize efficiencies, reduce the burden of redundancy, and leverage the potential to benefit both global and national public health by ensuring effective and efficient access to safe and effective quality medicines. To this end, the committee formulated five recommendations in the following areas:

- Improving public health through better-designed MRAs,
- Responding to evolving science and technology,
- Better utilization of the European Union (EU)-US MRA,
- Facilitating information sharing among international medicines regulators, and
- Evaluating public health impacts of recognition and reliance arrangements for medicines regulation.

IMPROVING PUBLIC HEALTH THROUGH BETTER-DESIGNED MRAs

Challenge

Most MRAs reference public health and safety. Article 2 of the EU-US MRA specifically states the following goal: "facilitate trade and benefit public health by allowing each Party to leverage and to reallocate its inspection resources, including by avoiding duplication of inspections, so as to improve oversight of manufacturing facilities and better address quality risk and prevent adverse health consequences." Thus, while the EU-US MRA has a public health goal, the agreement was developed under the auspices of trade negotiations, with trade facilitation featuring prominently in the discussions.

A shift in focus to public health would change the perspective, driving MRAs toward the goal of improved public health with an emphasis on patients. Furthermore, the type of arrangement a regulatory body chose to explore could be guided by public health goals specific to the needs of its jurisdiction.

Opportunity

The most formal information-sharing arrangements between medicines regulators have typically been legally binding MRAs, in which one agency recognizes the work and actions of another as equivalent to its own and something it can rely on. In discussions regarding MRAs and other regulatory reliance arrangements, it is essential that the goals of international commerce and freer trade not be pursued at the expense of improved public health for either party involved. To the contrary, as discussed above, advancing public health for all concerned must be the focus when these arrangements are designed, developed, and implemented.

Opportunity: Ensuring that meeting public health needs is the primary mission of MRAs and other reliance agreements requires that these agreements are designed with goals of advancing public health and these agreements are primarily designed, developed, and implemented by medicines regulators.

Recommendation 2: Policy makers, including lawmakers, should explore empowering regulators to expand the scope and substance of future mutual recognition agreements (MRAs) that address issues related to the safety, efficacy, and manufacturing quality of medicines, and to ensure that these MRAs are designed, developed, and imple-

mented primarily by medicines regulators. Policy makers will also need to ensure that regulators have adequate resources for these tasks.[1]

RESPONDING TO EVOLVING SCIENCE AND TECHNOLOGY

Challenge

The challenge of responding to evolving science and technology is related to the challenge, delineated below, regarding the scope of the EU-US MRA. The current EU-US MRA applies to GMP inspections of a limited range of medicine types. In addition, it mandates that the Joint Committee (Art. 20) consider the inclusion of veterinary medicines, vaccines for human use, plasma-derived pharmaceuticals (i.e., albumin, coagulation factors, and immunoglobulins), and clinical trial material for investigational products.[2] However, this expansion would remain limited to GMP inspections.

Challenge: As currently designed, MRAs are not sufficiently agile tools to respond to the rapid pace at which science and technology are evolving.

Opportunity

Both the EU and the United States have approval pathways for biosimilars. Since the United States first approved the pathway in 2010, 17 biosimilars have been approved, only 7 of which have made it to the market, primarily because of ongoing patent disputes (Zhai et al., 2019). In contrast, since 2006, EMA has approved 59 biosimilar applications, and it currently has 53 biosimilars available for sale in the EU (Harston, 2019).

Opportunity: More agile reliance arrangements would be better suited to meet the challenges posed by rapidly evolving science and technology. Allowing regulators to develop such arrangements would enhance global public health.

---

[1]Murray Lumpkin, Lembit Rago, and Katherine Bond did not fully concur with this recommendation because they believe it still leaves the negotiation, oversight, and finalization of MRAs related to medicines regulation to trade negotiators, rather than empowering medicines regulators to design, develop, conclude, and implement these specific medicines regulatory MRAs on their own. They believe that is the only way to ensure that public health is the sole focus of the negotiation and agreement and that the agreement is negotiated and concluded in the collaborative public health atmosphere that exists among medicines regulators and not the competitive business dynamic that pervades and shades trade negotiations.

[2]United States-European Union Amended Sectoral Annex for Pharmaceutical Good Manufacturing Practices (GMP), Article 20, Paragraph 2.

Thus, to address the public health challenges of the globalized production of medicines, as well as the growing need to address the medicine requirements during public health emergencies, the committee believes that MRAs and other reliance arrangements should be expanded to include new areas.

Recommendation 3: The committee recommends that regulators consider increasing the current scope of both formal and less formal reliance arrangements, including mutual recognition agreements, and that policy makers encourage regulatory authorities to explore formal and informal opportunities for reliance arrangements with other trusted regulatory authorities that give regulators greater flexibility in responding to challenges that affect their responsibility in overseeing the quality, safety, and efficacy of medicines throughout the medicines' lifecycle. Potential areas identified for such expansion of scope include good laboratory practice, good clinical practice, and good pharmacovigilance practice inspection reports; preclinical assessment reports; bioequivalence assessment reports; and a wider scope of product classes covered by such arrangements.

BETTER UTILIZATION OF THE EU-US MRA

Challenge

As discussed previously, formal and informal (bilateral and multilateral) reliance arrangements have the potential to improve public health protection through increased sharing of information and the reallocation of resources for the inspection of drug manufacturing facilities with potentially higher public health risks (FDA, 2019b). In 2008, following the discovery of contaminated heparin originating from China, the Bush administration announced provisions that would allow U.S. regulators to coordinate certain product manufacturing inspections with Australian and European regulators in China and India, setting the stage for so-called "third-country" inspections (i.e., inspections conducted outside of a regulator's jurisdiction). This was a critical step in addressing the rapid globalization of medicines production. The 2-year International API Inspection Pilot Programme reported overall positive results, having "contributed substantially to a better understanding of regional approaches to inspection and the building of mutual confidence" (EMA, 2011).

Sharing the results of inspections carried out in third countries is an integral part of the MRA between the EU and Switzerland. That MRA was amended in 2017 to include sharing of results of inspections (conducted by the Parties to the MRA) in third countries and batch certification if a product originates from a third-country manufacturer inspected by either Swiss or European regulators (EMA, 2018a). (See Chapter 3 for information on batch certification.) Such reliance on inspections of manufacturers located in third countries is critical in regions where overseas inspections have proven difficult because of operational challenges, and where the number of facilities needing inspection is very large and historically has exceeded the resources available for such inspections.

However, the sharing of information from inspection reports of third-country manufacturers is, at present, inefficient. Efficiency would be improved by the development of better mechanisms for sharing that information, coordination of inspections to avoid duplication, and joint identification and prioritizing of high-risk sites for inspections. Demonstrating the value of such coordination and information sharing could further strengthen trust among regulatory agencies charged with implementing the EU-US MRA, which includes a provision to share results of inspections in third countries. Doing so could potentially expand the range of oversight in countries with less rigorous regulatory oversight. In addition, the EU-US MRA was written to include only nine marketed products in the form of tablets, capsules, ointments, or injectables while excluding human blood and plasma, human tissues and organs, and advanced-therapy medicinal products (EMA, 2019f). (Vaccines and medicines derived from plasma are expected to be added to the MRA list by 2022.) Expanding the scope of the EU-US MRA could make better use of that agreement for purposes of public health protection.

> *Challenge: The EU-US MRA, as currently written, narrowly applies only to areas involving GMP and only to a limited range of products. Even so, some of its provisions have not been implemented.*

Opportunity

A decade after the heparin scare of 2008, concerns about ensuring the quality of APIs and finished pharmaceutical products from China and India continue. In 2018, FDA announced a voluntary recall of some generic medications used to treat high blood pressure and heart disease (FDA, 2018a). Between 2018 and 2019, FDA sent 75 warning letters, roughly half of which went to pharmaceutical manufacturers in China and India (Wilkinson, 2019). The EU also issued notices of noncompliance, roughly two-thirds of which were directed to medicines manufacturers in China and India (Wilkinson, 2019). MRAs and other reliance arrangements among trusted regulatory authorities would allow them to avoid duplicative inspections at sites demonstrating compliant GMP and to focus on sites that have not been inspected or that are in need of re-inspection following noncompliance. The provision in the EU-US MRA for inspections (conducted by the Parties to the MRA) in third countries, if implemented, could further extend the reach of both agencies.

As noted, MRAs cover primarily GMP and batch certification, although a few also include GLP. The inclusion of both GLP and GCP represents an opportunity to expand present MRAs to go beyond GMP inspections (i.e., manufacturing and production) to include assessment reports related to generics and biosimilars, as well as new medicines. To progress beyond GMP, however, MRA regulators would likely have to demonstrate high levels of trust and confidence by building a track record of demonstrated equivalence.

Opportunity: The provisions in the EU-US MRA for inspections conducted outside of the respective territories, which have not yet been implemented, could be implemented immediately. The EU-US MRA could be expanded to go beyond GMP to other regulatory activities, together with greater product coverage.

If one MRA regulatory authority can trust the other to perform an inspection within the latter authority's own jurisdiction, the committee could find no reason to doubt the ability of the latter authority to perform a quality inspection outside its own jurisdiction—especially as these inspections are currently limited to surveillance inspections. The EU-US MRA could be expanded to go beyond its currently limited GMP focus to a broader GMP focus and to other regulatory activities, together with greater product coverage.

Recommendation 4: Regulatory authorities in the United States and the European Union (EU) should immediately implement provisions included in the current EU-US mutual recognition agreement (MRA) (e.g., those regarding so-called "third-country" good manufacturing practice [GMP] inspections). Regulatory authorities also should begin considering the potential for expanding the EU-US MRA to include reliance in areas beyond GMP and a broader scope of products under the current GMP provisions.

FACILITATING INFORMATION SHARING AMONG INTERNATIONAL MEDICINES REGULATORS

Challenge

The questions of how, when, if, and to what extent regulatory agencies can share commercial confidential information and trade secrets is a very real concern for industry. Companies do not want their trade secrets (e.g., product manufacturing processes and chemical formulations) shared, given their fear that this could result in the theft of their intellectual and physical property with no compensation. Accordingly, regulatory authorities sometimes err on the side of excessive caution and redact inspection and other reports so as to protect confidential information and trade secrets and minimize their liability (Schwartz, 2017). While these fears do have a basis in some cases, however, they are not relevant in other cases, when a company has already submitted the same information to another regulator for its review.

The usability of a report diminishes significantly if, as a consequence of redaction, one regulator is unable to sufficiently understand another's report to fully grasp what occurred, what the other agency's assessments were, and on what they were based. Without such complete understanding, the agency seeking to rely on another agency's assessment is often left with little choice but to do its own full assessment or inspection to make a truly fully informed regulatory decision. TGA, for example, requires that unredacted reports be submitted by any sponsor seeking rapid approval using TGA's "comparable overseas regulators" processes for prescription medicines. The agencies from which TGA will accept unredacted reports include Health Canada, the Health Science Authority in Singapore, Swissmedic, the United Kingdom's Medicines & Healthcare products Regulatory Agency, FDA, and EMA (TGA, 2018). In Switzerland, it is up to the companies involved to provide for their medicinal products unredacted reports that are identical to those submitted and authorized abroad. Redacted reports are accepted, but the process is significantly slower, and thus higher fees are often imposed (Swissmedic, Form Information for application Art. 13 TPA HMV4, 03.02.2019). FDA has traditionally shared only heavily redacted reports (Schwartz, 2017), and regulatory partners wishing to rely on FDA inspection reports have been unable to do so because of these numerous redactions (Schwartz, 2017).

One of the goals of MRAs and other reliance arrangements is to decrease or eliminate duplicative inspections; heavy redaction impedes this goal. In addition to being costly, unnecessary duplicative clinical research trials pose ethical dilemmas, as patient participants may be exposed to undue distress (physical, emotional, etc.) or be considered ineligible for other clinical trials that could improve their health, while the duplicative trial offers little or no benefit for the public health community (Myles et al., 2014; Paquette et al., 2019). As part of the recent MRA with the EU, FDA has indicated it will begin sharing unredacted reports with its equivalent, trusted partner through the super confidentiality commitment (Super-CC) (EC, 2017). This shift in thinking for FDA has the potential to pave the way for future pilots with equally trusted regulatory authority partners. How many potential partners this might include is uncertain, but under current approaches, it is not thought to be more than a handful. Whether the current approach to redaction is a relevant good regulatory and good public health practice in a 21st-century world of globalized product development, production, distribution, and use is a question worth rethinking.

In the above context, the committee identified the following challenge with respect to open and transparent information sharing between regulatory partners.

> *Challenge: Regulators with recognized technical capacity and harmonized interests currently experience needless challenges in sharing complete information on which other regulators can rely to inform their own decision making. When regulators receive incomplete information from other regulators, they often must use their limited resources to needlessly repeat inspections or data assessments.*

Opportunity

There is great value in reading and being able to use other regulators' inspection reports (Roth et al., 2018), especially when these reports are from regulators with recognized technical capacity and harmonized interests. First, for those less familiar with inspection processes, knowledge is gained by seeing how an inspection was conducted, what areas were covered, and how the findings were documented. Second, trust is built through the willful sharing of complete information. History shows that trust can lead to reliance pilots, which, if successful, can be elevated even further to more substantive collaborative arrangements. Third, the information gained by reviewing the findings of others' inspection reports allows regulators to make more informed sovereign decisions, most often without having to use their own limited resources to perform what would be a redundant inspection exercise. Each of these benefits, based on greater transparency and completeness of inspection reports, helps strengthen the global public health infrastructure for safe and effective quality medicines through learning and greater insights into what manufacturers are actually doing. By offering helpful inspection reports that regulators around the world can view, regulatory bodies with recognized technical capacity and harmony of interests can facilitate the robustness of other regulators' decision making.

Currently, EMA offers a public assessment report with only commercially confidential material redacted,[3] and FDA is running a pilot program—with nine companies' new drug applications—assessing the feasibility of

---

[3]Regulation (EC) No 726/2004 of the European Parliament and of the Council of 31 March 2004 laying down community procedures for the authorization and supervision of medicinal products for human and veterinary use and establishing a European Medicines Agency.

publicly releasing portions of clinical study reports. The goal of this pilot is to enhance public

> understanding of information about drug approvals to improve the accuracy of discussions about drug approvals in scientific publications, increasing stakeholders' understanding of the basis for FDA's approval decisions, and informing physicians and other health care providers about the clinical trial results on which regulatory decisions are based. (FDA, 2019a, p. 30734).

Both efforts indicate the willingness by regulators and industry to share information for the public good, although impediments still remain with respect to providing more transparent and complete assessment and inspection reports throughout all phases of a product's lifecycle. Regulators must balance a desire to provide other regulators with access to unredacted inspection reports against the need to honor the legal requirements for protecting "trade secrets and commercial or financial information which is privileged or confidential."[4]

Opportunity: Increasing information sharing and the transparency of each other's regulatory activities can facilitate medicines regulators' more efficient resource allocation and decision making. Making complete/unredacted assessment and inspection information available to other regulators will enable more equitable access to quality regulatory information for a greater number of regulatory authorities to address global public health needs.

The committee identified three areas within this opportunity:

Sharing of Inspection Reports

- Sharing of complete unredacted inspection reports would facilitate learning, aid in decision making, reduce the use of limited resources on redundant inspections, and strengthen the overall global public heath infrastructure for safe and effective quality medicines.
- The benefits of sharing complete unredacted inspection reports could be enhanced by aligning the formats of the reports to facilitate information exchange and increase the reports' value to the receiving authorities, thereby enabling learning and sovereign decision making by regulatory authorities with fewer resources. (For example, the Pharmaceutical Inspection Co-operation Scheme format for inspection reports could be a starting point for such

[4] 21 CFR § 20.61.

alignment.) This benefit is predicated on the sponsor's intent to market the exact same version of the product that was authorized and inspected by the agency on which the receiving agency is relying. Shipping an alternative (e.g., "rest of world") version manufactured in a different plant or on a different manufacturing line would negate the ability to rely on the inspection reports of a reliable counterpart.

Sharing of Assessment Reports

- Without a unified platform and a standard format for reporting, the sharing of assessment, inspection, and other reports can be challenging. An opportunity exists for regulators to freely share these reports in a standardized format with other regulators with whom legally authorized appropriate confidentiality arrangements exist.
- Where the above arrangements do not exist, sponsors could explicitly allow regulators to share full assessment reports on specified products with particular regulators.

FDA Information Sharing

- The Super-CC includes medicines, providing a mechanism for FDA to share unredacted information with regulatory authorities under very specific circumstances. The opportunity exists for FDA to ensure that current redaction practices optimize information sharing consistent with current law and for Congress to reevaluate whether existing confidentiality restrictions are still fit-for-purpose in the 21st-century globalized environment in which these products exist.

Without a unified platform and a standard format for reporting, the sharing of assessment and inspection reports can be challenging. The committee recognized that some regulators currently share assessment, inspection, and other reports with other regulators with whom legally authorized appropriate confidentiality arrangements exist. In instances where they do not exist, sponsors could explicitly allow regulators to share full assessment reports on specified products with particular regulators. Additionally, the Super-CC between FDA and the EU includes medicines. The Super-CC provides a mechanism for FDA to share essentially unredacted information with regulatory authorities under very specific circumstances.

The committee believes that to best meet the public health goals of reliance arrangements, an opportunity exists for FDA and Congress to ensure that current redaction practices optimize information sharing. To this end, FDA and Congress could reevaluate whether existing confidentiality restrictions are still fit-for-purpose in the 21st-century globalized environment in which these products exist and whether modifications are needed to meet the public health goals for these arrangements noted earlier in this report (e.g., protecting and promoting public health; reducing the burden of regulatory redundancy on patients, industry, and regulators; allowing regulators to use the finite human and financial resources they currently have most effectively and efficiently; and helping to bring needed quality medicines to patients domestically and globally as efficiently as possible).

Recommendation 5: Regulatory authorities, with guidance from their governmental leaders, should undertake determining whether current limitations on sharing regulatory work products with other regulatory authorities are still fit-for-purpose to help protect and promote public health; to reduce the burden of regulatory redundancy on patients, industry, and regulators; to allow regulators globally to best utilize the limited technical and financial resources currently available to them to meet their public health mandates; and to bring needed quality medicines to patients domestically and globally as efficiently as possible.

EVALUATING PUBLIC HEALTH IMPACTS OF RECOGNITION AND RELIANCE ARRANGEMENTS FOR MEDICINES REGULATION

Challenge

Recognition and reliance arrangements have been operational over varied timeframes, some for as long as two decades, and in a variety of different contexts. Accordingly, they could offer lessons as to what the most successful such arrangements have in common and their short-, medium-, and long-term benefits. However, such lessons could not be supported by evidence because of a dearth of data.

Furthermore, a review of the texts of such arrangements indicates that most do not explicitly call for evaluation of direct or indirect health benefits, although a few do contain language on monitoring the implementation and functioning of the arrangement itself. For example, the New Zealand Trans-Tasman Mutual Recognition Agreement incorporates a "general review" of the arrangement's operations at given time intervals (TTMRA § 12.1.1). This review is intended to "assess the effectiveness of the arrangements in fostering and enhancing trade and workforce mobility between Australia and New Zealand and an assessment of any amendments or additions" (TTMRA § 12.1.2).

In 1995, FDA finalized its Compliance Policy Guide pertaining to international agreements (CPG Sec. 100.900, "International Memoranda of Understanding," updated March 2, 2015). This guide lays out considerations for entering into international agreements and delineates the reasons for doing so, including (1) benefits to health (the potential for "risk reduction associated with products or programs," prioritization of "products imported into the United States," risk-based assessment ["history of compliance problems"]); (2) the "regulatory burden on industry"; and (3) the "U.S. foreign policy objectives and priorities of other U.S. government agencies."

It is worth noting that since the 1990s, Drug Master Files[5] from India and China have increased markedly compared with those of the United States and the EU. More broadly, as discussed previously, the supply chain for medicines has become more complex as a result of the globalization of manufacturing and production. Such considerations as risks associated with the globalized supply chain and rapidly developing novel treatments and innovative products that were relevant in 2019 were not explicitly among the considerations laid out in 1995 (Chace-Ortiz, 2017).

Anecdotally, regulators who have had experience with MRAs report benefits to these agreements, but those benefits are not quantified. Informational interviews conducted for this study revealed the potential benefits or pointed to potential measurable outcomes (see the discussion in the "Opportunity" section below). At the time of this writing, the EU-US MRA was too recent to have been evaluated. Nevertheless, the committee was advised by FDA that a benefit/cost analysis of the MRA was planned.

> *Challenge: Evaluating effects of recognition and reliance arrangements on public health, use of resources, and essential regulatory competencies is challenging because of a dearth of frameworks, metrics, and data for use in such evaluations. The texts of existing formal and less formal reliance arrangements fail to incorporate review criteria or frameworks, including specific metrics, by which regulatory authorities and the broader community could evaluate the arrangements' public health impacts.*

Opportunity

The Government Performance and Results Act of 1993 (Pub. L. No. 103-62) and successor legislation (GPRA Modernization Act of 2010, Pub. L. No. 111-352) mandated that federal agencies set goals, measure results,

[5] A Drug Master File is a submission to FDA that may be used to provide confidential detailed information about facilities, processes, or articles used in the manufacturing, processing, packaging, and storing of one or more human drugs. See https://www.fda.gov/drugs/forms-submission-requirements/drug-master-files-dmfs (accessed September 28, 2019).

and report progress. Relatedly, the Foundations for Evidence-Based Policymaking Act of 2018 (Pub. L. No. 115-435) "requires agency data to be accessible and requires agencies to plan to develop statistical evidence to support policymaking."

Currently, assessment of reliance arrangements globally is generally focused on agreement monitoring rather than on public health objectives per se. Results-based frameworks are utilized increasingly in the public sector and international organizations to shift the focus of monitoring and evaluation from processes to results (Zall Kusek and Rist, 2004). These frameworks reflect a theory of change in a logical fashion (i.e., in the spirit of "What gets measured gets done") and incorporate planning for results monitoring and measurement into the organization. Within the past decade, FDA has introduced results frameworks to address various aspects of its import safety and inspection programs. The committee anticipates that this focus on public health results rather than agreement monitoring will better further public health goals consistent with the agency's broader mission.

OECD (Correia de Brito et al., 2016) has identified three potential public health benefits of MRAs: (1) managing risks and externalities across borders, (2) achieving greater administrative efficiency, and (3) improving knowledge flow and peer learning among regulators. OECD (2013a) conducted a review of the literature assessing the empirical evidence for these public health benefits and found it comparatively sparse in comparison with the evidence on economic gains.

The committee's interviews with regulators pointed to potential outcome measures that would reflect the public health benefits of recognition and reliance arrangements, although those benefits are not yet being measured. These potential outcome measures included number of inspections in higher-risk areas, number of sites inspected for the first time, redeployment of staff to higher-risk product areas and regions, and rapid response to alerts and incidents involving GMP noncompliance. Regulators noted that such collaborative activities as joint training programs on GMP and GCP were relatively easy to quantify as outputs of agreements.

High-quality assessments can prompt substantial improvements in an agency's ability to fulfill its surveillance duties. For example, the U.S. Government Accountability Office (GAO) has been closely monitoring the overseas work of FDA since having issued its first assessment report on FDA's international work in medicines regulation in 2008 (GAO, 2008). At that time, policy makers recognized the intense challenges faced by FDA as a result of globalization in ensuring for U.S. consumers safe and effective medicines coming from various parts of the world. FDA responded with a wide array of initiatives, including a joint inspections pilot project with EU regulators and the International API Inspection Pilot Programme, mentioned previously, whereby regulators from the EU and Australia would share plans to inspect, as well as inspection results from API manufacturing sites. Both initiatives were meant to build trust and confidence between regulatory bodies. In particular, the information-sharing activity has helped regulators use their resources more efficiently by minimizing overlap in their inspection scheduling plans.

Assessments may also impact the quality and effectiveness of enforcement actions. For example, GAO's 2016 report on FDA's overseas progress in drug safety noted two performance measures used by FDA to assess its foreign offices in ensuring drug safety: (1) number of foreign inspections and (2) number of collaborative actions (GAO, 2016).[6] GAO identified weaknesses in the latter measure with respect to drug safety, as the annual target of 25 collaborative actions did not specify commodity, was not unique to the foreign offices, and could not easily be tied to an outcome involving drug safety. Furthermore, GAO pointed to activities undertaken that could surface drug safety outcomes not included in the measures. An example cited by GAO referenced intelligence gathered from FDA's office in India regarding fraudulent APIs manufactured in that country, resulting in death in another country. FDA staff in India followed up to determine inspection results of the local government, and upon confirmation of noncompliance with clinical GMP, the agency placed the company and its affiliate on import alert.

Recent assessments have highlighted additional opportunities to enhance surveillance through better international reliance. A 2019 GAO *High Risk Series* report included an update on FDA's international oversight of medicines (GAO, 2019). In that update, GAO suggested that FDA develop more fully its measures for tracking how overseas offices contribute to drug safety outcomes. The report also applauded FDA's progress in responding to present-day medicines regulatory challenges through a variety of interventions that included signing the MRA with the European Commission. As discussed earlier, this MRA, which became fully functional in July 2019, includes provisions[7] for formally accepting third-country inspections conducted by the other region's regulatory bodies.[8] That is, under the current MRA, the United States and the EU could accept inspec-

[6] "FDA defines a collaborative action as concrete regulatory and public health actions, or initiatives that contribute toward supporting OIP objectives and outcomes" (GAO, 2016, p. 26).

[7] Art. 8.3: "A Party may accept official GMPs documents issued by a recognized authority of the other Party for manufacturing facilities located outside the territory of the issuing authority." See http://trade.ec.europa.eu/doclib/docs/2017/february/tradoc_155398.pdf (accessed September 28, 2019).

[8] Annex to the Commission Decision on determining the Union position for a Decision of the Joint Committee set up under Article 14 of the Agreement on Mutual Recognition between the European Community and the United States, in order to amend the Sectoral Annex on Pharmaceutical Good Manufacturing Practices.

tion reports accepted by each other's agencies concerning a manufacturing plant not located in the EU or the United States. Currently, the implementation of the EU-US MRA has in scope only EU inspections performed in the EU and FDA inspections performed in the United States.

> **Recommendation 6: When formal and informal recognition and reliance arrangements are being developed, the regulatory authorities involved should co-create a results framework with clear indicators/metrics and processes for monitoring and measuring the arrangements' results and impacts to enhance understanding of their public health and other benefits and associated regulatory efficiencies, and enable benefit/risk and cost/benefit analysis of the arrangements over time.**

6

The Way Forward

Given the structure of the Statement of Task for this study, much of the committee's work focused on mutual recognition agreements (MRAs) and thus concentrated heavily on recognition and reliance within good manufacturing practice (GMP). However, the committee recognized the critical importance of other aspects of regulation across the lifecycle of a medicine. In particular, the committee believes public health would benefit greatly from more regulatory cooperation in the area of medicines safety and suggests further exploration by regulatory authorities and other stakeholders within the areas of pharmacovigilance (PV) and post-market surveillance.

PHARMACOVIGILANCE AND POST-MARKET SURVEILLANCE

PV can be distinguished from post-market surveillance as follows. The World Health Organization (WHO, 2019a) defines PV as "the science and activities relating to the detection, assessment, understanding and prevention of adverse effects or any other drug-related problem." This means monitoring for safety across the entire lifecycle of the medicine. In contrast, as the name implies, post-market surveillance is directed at safety issues occurring only after a medicine has reached the market. Post-market surveillance is an essential step in better ensuring the safety of medicines because, unlike the controlled environment of a clinical trial, it represents "real life" situations in which patients may differ from the populations used in the drug approval study, and in which consumption of other medicines and lifestyle choices could affect how a medicine is metabolized within a person or population. Post-market surveillance also encompasses good storage and distribution practices (WHO, 2019b) and field surveillance activities to assess the quality of a product on the market.

Given the globalization of the pharmaceutical industry, it stands to reason that greater regulatory cooperation could benefit patients in multiple jurisdictions; however, differences across countries in the areas of PV regulations, systems, and processes place limitations on such cooperation (Hans and Gupta, 2018). A general trend away from reactive ("passive") PV approaches and toward proactive ("active") PV approaches may open an opportunity for establishing systems for greater sharing of safety information and data in the post-market phase. The European Union (EU) is an example of this evolution. There is now a unified database, known as EudraVigilance, where manufacturers, patients, and care providers can submit adverse drug reaction reports (EMA, 2019a). In this way, the European Medicines Agency and member states' regulatory authorities can monitor the safety of medicines for timely detection and assessment of safety signals. The U.S. Food and Drug Administration (FDA) has a similar system—the FDA Adverse Event Reporting System—whereby providers and consumers can submit information directly to FDA, while manufacturers are required to send any adverse event reports they receive (FDA, 2018c). The same is true for the EU.

Countries with well-developed PV systems often engage industry in taking a significant role in reporting to their regulatory authority, whereas other countries with less developed systems may use hospitals or universities as regional PV centers for collecting and analyzing reports on adverse reactions to medicines (Dal Pan, 2014). Monitoring of adverse events is typically supplemented by a process of routine inspections of facilities along with sampling and testing of medicines. In remarks to the committee (July 10, 2019), Emer Cooke, head of medicines regulation at WHO, offered a series of suggestions for adding emphasis on reliance in the post-approval phase that could help stimulate dialogue among stakeholders moving forward. These suggestions included

- proactively sharing post-market safety data;
- establishing standards for timeliness and minimum information content for posting emergent safety issues or regulatory actions;
- standardizing good pharmacovigilance practice (GPvP), including roles and responsibilities of industry in collecting and reporting foreign safety data; and
- encouraging reliance/work sharing throughout a product's lifecycle, in the monitoring of PV, manufacturing quality, and post-authorization safety and efficacy.

AGGREGATE SAFETY REPORTS

While individual case safety reports, as just described, provide valuable information on adverse events (e.g., potential adverse reactions) experienced by individuals, aggregate safety reports offer a broader profile of the medicine and its use in different populations (Kulkarni and Kulkarni, 2019). Based on these worldwide safety reports, safety signals can be generated, further confirmatory data can be generated if needed, and medicine labels can then be updated in accordance with the findings that optimize the safe use of the medicine. The International Council for Harmonisation of Technical Requirements for Pharmaceuticals for Human Use-standard Periodic Safety Update Report (PSUR) is a tool used by many agencies and companies around the world for post-authorization benefit/risk analysis of a medicine. PSURs are composed by the marketing authorization holder (i.e., the company/sponsor)—using the Periodic Benefit/Risk Evaluation Reports (PBRERs) format—and submitted to the appropriate regulatory authority at predetermined time points. Like the PSUR, the harmonized PBRER "is intended to promote a consistent approach to periodic postmarketing safety reporting among the ICH regions and to enhance efficiency by reducing the number of reports generated for submission to regulatory authorities" (FDA, 2016, p. 3). In the United States, Periodic Adverse Drug Experience Reports are submitted to FDA for safety monitoring of medicines with market approval in this country, although waivers are given so that global PSURs/PBRERs can be submitted if they contain the information FDA has requested.

EXPANDING MUTUAL RECOGNITION AGREEMENTS TO GO BEYOND GOOD MANUFACTURING PRACTICE

In Recommendation 4 in Chapter 5, the committee encourages regulatory authorities in the United States and in the EU to consider "the potential for expanding the EU-US MRA to include reliance in areas beyond GMP and a broader scope of products under the current GMP provisions." The committee was intentional in this wording. The committee saw no drawbacks in "considering the potential," nor did it hear negative comments about expanding the scope of recognition and reliance throughout the information gathering for this study. Although the committee initially acknowledged possible fears of reduced human and financial resources and a loss of sovereignty due to greater reliance, none of those fears were substantiated in any of its information-gathering interviews. To the contrary, it became apparent to the committee that even MRAs (and the other, less formal arrangements) preserve sovereign decision making and have not adversely affected resources. At the same time, despite the value of MRAs for achieving greater reliance between regulators, the committee came to realize that formal trade-orientated MRAs may not be the best vehicle for medicines regulatory activities; rather, formal and informal recognition and reliance arrangements designed, developed, agreed upon, and implemented by medicines regulators would be the most appropriate way forward (see Recommendation 2 in Chapter 5).

In contemplating potential areas for MRA expansion, the committee identified as worthy of consideration GCP reports, GLP reports, GPvP reports, and reviews of PSURs. Consideration might be given to possibilities for sharing of reports or work-sharing arrangements with standardization of both the content and timing ("periodicity") of reports so regulatory agencies would receive the same reports at the same time. Another possibility for exploration might be in the pre-approval phase, with sharing of bioequivalence reports from generic drug firms submitting the exact same product in both countries—especially if the design is a three-arm design that uses both the EU- and the U.S.-listed reference product along with the test product. Pharmaceutical companies would likely be attracted to the idea of one review used by both agencies, and perhaps this could help alleviate some of the medicines shortages in both jurisdictions.

With regard to other products that the EU-US MRA might expand to encompass, some thought could first be given to biologics, perhaps starting with well-characterized biologics such as monoclonals, and then vaccines. Veterinary products were not part of this committee's charge, which covered only human medicines, but in considering the expansion of MRA implementation, some thought might go into implementing the existing provision for animal medicines. For more distant consideration, collaborative arrangements between the two regulatory authorities in reviewing such innovations as gene therapies and some newer cutting-edge modalities might also be explored.

EVALUATING PUBLIC HEALTH IMPACTS OF RECOGNITION AND RELIANCE

The committee looked at its sixth recommendation (see Chapter 5) as an opportunity for regulatory authorities to work together in co-creating a public health results framework and metrics, at the same time an agreement is being developed. However, the committee also recognized the difficulties associated with quantitatively measuring improved public health. At some point, the public health benefit is inferred and/or intuitive. This is not to say that quantitative and qualitative measures should not be collected, however. Rather, public health indicators should be collected based on the up-front, agreed-upon intent of the arrangement. For example, if better utilization of resources is a goal, perhaps there could be some specific metrics around whether resources were being better utilized. The result of the use of this measure might be to learn that because of this agreement, X number of inspectors had been redeployed from an area of low to high risk, or an increase of X number of manufacturing sites, including new or high-risk sites, had been inspected. These numbers would then be extrapolated to imply a public health impact. Such measurements would go beyond simply affirming that certain activities had been undertaken, to now considering how the undertaking of those activities compared with the status quo before the agreement was implemented.

In the committee's vision, such measurements would be agreement-specific. While it may be impractical to propose a global framework given the specific nature of recognition and reliance arrangements, the committee was intrigued by the idea of regulators agreeing upon a key set of metrics reflecting a more global public health approach. A global-level conversation could be led by a group such as the International Coalition of Medicines Regulatory Authorities (ICMRA), involving the chief executive officers of the major medicines regulatory agencies globally, that addresses regulatory science issues through enhanced communication and information sharing among regulators. The discussions might include such questions as what "good" looks like under these arrangements, how an agency knows whether the benefits of an arrangement outweigh its (internal) costs, and what parameters might be reported annually so that the agencies and other stakeholders can better understand what is occurring under the auspices of the arrangement.

In addition to ICMRA, WHO—in relation to its planned Good Reliance Practices Guidelines—might be another group to develop some global metrics for these arrangements, particularly if metrics were proposed for measuring the impact of implementing Good Reliance Practices in an annex to the guidelines. The committee believes that even if the proposed metrics were not detailed or comprehensive, some high-level principles and good examples would likely be helpful in structuring future work in this area.

FINAL THOUGHTS

It is the committee's hope that its landscaping of the medicines regulatory environment will better position regulators, policy makers, and technical and public health experts to address some of the 21st-century challenges facing national leaders around the world in ensuring safe and effective medicines for their countries' people. As outlined in Chapter 2, these challenges range from ramifications of globalization, to drug shortages, to disease outbreaks. Each of these challenges calls for responses whose central focus is the public's health. Chapter 5 provides the committee's conclusion and recommendations based on key opportunities, including a strategy for mounting responses that largely reflects messages from a wide array of stakeholders who provided input for this study, as well as the committee's own knowledge of and expertise in medicines regulation. All of the opportunities outlined in Chapter 5 are built on a foundation of trust, confidence, and reliance within a collaborative dynamic. For example, interactions through working groups and other informal activities often begin the process of building trusted relationships that help establish confidence in the work of other regulators. As trust and confidence grow, they can lead to pilot activities whereby regulators test their ability to rely on each other's work to inform their own decision making. Such reliance further increases trust and confidence among the partners, who may then agree to acknowledge their reliance more formally, such as through an MRA in which a higher degree of reliance on the partner's decisions is acknowledged.

As regulators contemplate metrics with a public health focus, it would be wise to consider the views of patients and their desire for access to quality-assured, safe, and effective medicines. Patients are also interested in equity. Persons with rare diseases are acutely aware of the scarcity of study subjects needed for research and development of breakthrough medicines and the importance of working across national boundaries for the testing of new drugs. Speeding this process through greater regulatory cooperation across borders is something patients seek. These issues are what the public cares about, and a public health framing might consider such patient-centered perspectives in the design and evaluation of recognition and reliance arrangements.

Well-resourced regulatory agencies are well positioned to grapple with the challenges posed by continuing innovations in medicine and technology, such as gene therapies and other advanced therapeutics for regulators charged with ensuring the quality, safety, and efficacy of cutting-edge medicines. Nonetheless, shared access to specialists with expertise in highly technical product research, development, manufacturing, and production could help even the well-resourced regulatory agencies stay abreast of the rapidly evolving science of medicines. For lower-resourced authorities also struggling with this challenge—within a context of growing workloads and restricted resources and the limitations thereby imposed—considering the findings of well-resourced agencies and working collaboratively with these agencies might be a mechanism for bringing innovative products into their markets. This does not mean that all countries would automatically accept the findings of other agencies. As is the case today with many regulators, if such information were shared, each medicines regulatory authority could weigh the benefits and risks of approving a medicine for its country's people.

In the end, medicines regulatory authorities are required to demonstrate their ability to protect and promote the health of the people within their jurisdiction. Every regulatory authority faces this challenge while at the same time confronting the set of unique circumstances in which it functions. Access to financial and human resources is highly variable, as are population characteristics because of variations in genetics and environmental exposure to health risks, cultural practices, burdens of disease, social perspectives, health care systems, demographics, and societal income levels. Despite all of these differences, however, the tie that binds the work of all medicines regulators is their mandate to facilitate and help ensure the availability of quality-assured, safe, and effective medicines to serve the public health. It is the committee's firmly held belief that this mandate can be met through effective use of the full range of formal and informal recognition and reliance arrangements that preserve national interests while placing the public's health at the core of all regulatory efforts.

References

Ahonkhai, V., S. F. Martins, A. Portet, M. Lumpkin, and D. Hartman. 2016. Speeding access to vaccines and medicines in low- and middle-income countries: A case for change and a framework for optimized product market authorization. *PLOS ONE* 11(11):e0166515.

Andrade, E. L., A. Bento, J. Cavalli, S. K. Oliveira, R. C. Schwanke, J. M. Siqueira, C. S. Freitas, R. Marcon, and J. B. Calixto. 2016. Non-clinical studies in the process of new drug development—Part II: Good laboratory practice, metabolism, pharmacokinetics, safety and dose translation to clinical studies. *Brazilian Journal of Medical and Biological Research* 49(12). doi: 10.1590/1414-431X20165646.

APEC (Asia-Pacific Economic Cooperation). 2019. *Life sciences innovation forum.* https://www.apec.org/Groups/Committee-on-Trade-and-Investment/Life-Sciences-Innovation-Forum (accessed September 20, 2019).

Aronov, I. Z., A. M. Rybakova, V. Y. Salamatov, A. V. Tangaeva, and N. M. Galkina. 2019. Application of Chow test to estimate the effect of mutual recognition agreements. *International Journal of Mathematical, Engineering and Management Sciences* 4(3):591–600.

Babigumira, J., A. Stergachis, T. Kanyok, L. Evans, M. Hajjou, P. Nkansah, V. Pribluda, L. Garrison, and J. Nwokike. 2018. *A risk-based resource allocation framework for pharmaceutical quality assurance for medicines regulatory authorities in low- and middle-income countries.* Rockville, MD: US Pharmacopeial Convention.

Byrd, J. B., G. M. Chertow, and V. Bhalla. 2019. Hypertension hot potato—Anatomy of the angiotensin-receptor blocker recalls. *New England Journal of Medicine* 380(17):1589–1591.

Chace-Ortiz, M. 2017. The changing dynamics of global API manufacturing. *Chemica Oggi—Chemistry Today* 35:40–42.

Cooke, E. 2019. *WHO's Approaches to Promoting Reliance.* PowerPoint presention at the July 10–11, 2019, meeting of the Committee on Mutual Recognition Agreements and Reliance in the Regulation of Medicines, London, UK.

Correia de Brito, A., C. Kauffmann, and J. Pelkmans. 2016. *The contribution of mutual recognition to international regulatory co-operation.* OECD Regulatory Policy Working Paper No. 2. https://www.oecd.org/regreform/WP2_Contribution-of-mutual-recognition-to-IRC.pdf (accessed September 10, 2019).

Dal Pan, G. J. 2014. Ongoing challenges in pharmacovigilance. *Drug Safety* 37(1):1–8.

EC (European Commission). 2017. Pharmaceutical committee 27 October 2017 79th meeting. Summary Record. https://ec.europa.eu/health/sites/health/files/files/committee/pharm742_summary_record_final.pdf (accessed September 19, 2019).

EFPIA (European Federation of Pharmaceutical Industries and Associations). 2018. *Annual regulatory GMP/GDP inspection survey 2017 data*. https://www.efpia.eu/media/361849/_efpia-2017-reg-inspection-survey_public-summary.pdf (accessed September 18, 2019).

EMA (European Medicines Agency). 2009a. EMEA-FDA GCP initiative. General-EMEA/INS/GCP/541006/2008. https://www.ema.europa.eu/en/documents/other/european-medicines-agency-food-drug-administration-good-clinical-practice-initiative_en.pdf (accessed September 22, 2019).

EMA. 2009b. European Medicines Agency and U.S. Food and Drug Administration (FDA) launch good clinical practice initiative. Press Release. London, UK: EMA. https://www.ema.europa.eu/en/news/european-medicines-agency-us-food-drug-administration-fda-launch-good-clinical-practice-initiative (accessed September 18, 2019).

EMA. 2011. *Final report on the International API Inspection Pilot Programme*. https://www.ema.europa.eu/en/documents/report/final-report-international-active-pharmaceutical-ingredient-inspection-pilot-programme_en.pdf (accessed September 27, 2019).

EMA. 2013. *Mandate, objectives and rules of procedure: Good Clinical Practice Inspectors Working Group (GCP IWG)*. https://www.ema.europa.eu/en/documents/other/mandate-objectives-rules-procedure-gcp-inspectors-working-group-gcp-iwg_en.pdf (accessed September 19, 2019).

EMA. 2015. Europe to boost international cooperation on generics. News Release. https://www.ema.europa.eu/en/news/europe-boost-international-cooperation-generics (accessed September 23, 2019).

EMA. 2016. *Connecting the dots: Towards global knowledge of the international medicine regulatory landscape: Mapping of international initiatives*. https://www.ema.europa.eu/en/documents/leaflet/connecting-dots-towards-global-knowledge-international-medicine-regulatory-landscape-mapping_en.pdf (accessed September 12, 2019).

EMA. 2018a. *Annual report of the Good Manufacturing and Distribution Practice Inspectors Working Group 2017*. https://www.ema.europa.eu/en/documents/report/annual-report-good-manufacturing-distribution-practice-inspectors-working-group-2017_en.pdf (accessed September 18, 2019).

EMA. 2018b. *Report on the international active pharmaceutical ingredient inspection programme 2011–2016*. https://www.ema.europa.eu/en/documents/report/report-international-active-pharmaceutical-ingredient-api-inspection-programme-2011-2016_en.pdf (accessed September 20, 2019).

EMA. 2019a. *2018 Annual report on EudraVigilance for the European Parliament, the Council and the Commission. Reporting period: 1 January to 31 December 2018*. https://www.ema.europa.eu/en/documents/report/2018-annual-report-eudravigilance-european-parliament-council-commission-reporting-period-1-january_en.pdf (accessed September 20, 2019).

EMA. 2019b. Access to documents. https://www.ema.europa.eu/en/about-us/how-we-work/access-documents (accessed September 28, 2019).

EMA. 2019c. *Angiotensin-II-receptor antagonists (sartans) containing a tetrazole group*. https://www.ema.europa.eu/en/medicines/human/referrals/angiotensin-ii-receptor-antagonists-sartans-containing-tetrazole-group (accessed September 16, 2019).

EMA. 2019d. Bilateral interactions with non-EU regulators—China. https://www.ema.europa.eu/en/partners-networks/international-activities/bilateral-interactions-non-eu-regulators/china (accessed September 26, 2019).

EMA. 2019e. Cluster activities. https://www.ema.europa.eu/en/partners-networks/international-activities/cluster-activities (accessed September 29, 2019).

EMA. 2019f. Mutual recognition agreements (MRA). https://www.ema.europa.eu/en/human-regulatory/research-development/compliance/good-manufacturing-practice/mutual-recognition-agreements-mra (accessed September 2, 2019).

EMA. 2019g. Working parties and other groups. https://www.ema.europa.eu/en/committes/working-parties-other-groups (accessed September 4, 2019).

FDA (U.S. Food and Drug Administration). 1988. FDA–Netherlands, MOU regarding good laboratory practice. https://www.fda.gov/international-programs/cooperative-arrangements/fda-netherlands-mou-regarding-good-laboratory-practice (accessed September 16, 2019).

FDA. 2015a. *Manual of compliance policy guides*. https://www.fda.gov/inspections-compliance-enforcement-and-criminal-investigations/compliance-manuals/manual-compliance-policy-guides (accessed September 29, 2019).

FDA. 2015b. *Plan to increase access to results of FDA-funded scientific research*. https://www.fda.gov/media/90883/download (accessed September 10, 2019).

FDA. 2016. *Providing postmarketing periodic safety reports in the ICH E2C(R2) format (periodic benefit-risk evaluation report): Guidance for industry*. https://www.fda.gov/media/85520/download (accessed September 16, 2019).

FDA. 2017a. *Emergency use authorization of medical products and related authorities: Guidance for industry and other stakeholders*. https://www.fda.gov/regulatory-information/search-fda-guidance-documents/emergency-use-authorization-medical-products-and-related-authorities (accessed September 15, 2019).

FDA. 2017b. *Securing the future for Puerto Rico: Restoring the island's robust medical product manufacturing sector*. https://www.fda.gov/media/108975/download (accessed September 23, 2019).

FDA. 2018a. FDA announces voluntary recall of several medicines containing valsartan following detection of an impurity. Press Release. https://www.fda.gov/news-events/press-announcements/fda-announces-voluntary-recall-several-medicines-containing-valsartan-following-detection-impurity (accessed September 30, 2019).

FDA. 2018b. Foreign regulator information exchanges. https://www.fda.gov/vaccines-blood-biologics/international-activities/foreign-regulator-information-exchanges (accessed September 3, 2019).

FDA. 2018c. Questions and answers on FDA's adverse event reporting system (FAERS). https://www.fda.gov/drugs/surveillance/questions-and-answers-fdas-adverse-event-reporting-system-faers (accessed September 30, 2019).

FDA. 2018d. Statement by FDA Commissioner Scott Gottlieb, M.D., update on recovery efforts in Puerto Rico, and continued efforts to mitigate IV saline and amino acid drug shortages. Press Release. https://www.fda.gov/news-events/press-announcements/statement-fda-commissioner-scott-gottlieb-md-update-recovery-efforts-puerto-rico-and-continued (accessed September 30, 2019).

FDA. 2019a. E19 New drug regulatory program modernization: Improving approval package E documentation and communication. *Federal Register* 84(124):30733–30736.

FDA. 2019b. Mutual recognition agreement (MRA). https://www.fda.gov/international-programs/international-arrangements/mutual-recognition-agreement-mra (accessed August 18, 2019).

FDA. 2019c. *Report on drug shortages for calendar year 2018*. https://www.fda.gov/media/130561/download (accessed September 15, 2019).

GAO (U.S. Government Accountability Office). 2008. Better data management and more inspections are needed to strengthen FDA's foreign drug inspection program. News Release. https://www.gao.gov/new.items/d08970.pdf (accessed September 9, 2019).

GAO. 2016. FDA has improved its foreign drug inspection program, but needs to assess the effectiveness and staffing of its foreign offices. GAO Highlights. https://www.gao.gov/assets/690/681689.pdf (accessed September 9, 2019).

GAO. 2019. *Substantial efforts needed to achieve greater progress on high-risk areas.* https://www.gao.gov/assets/700/697245.pdf (accessed September 9, 2019).

Garbe, J. H. O., K. Ennis, G. M. Furer, M. G. Jacobs, and S. Rönninger. 2015. Import testing of pharmaceutical products has limited safety benefits and can add risk to patients. *Pharmaceutical Technology* 2015 Supplement(3):s18–s26.

Hans, M., and S. K. Gupta. 2018. Comparative evaluation of pharmacovigilance regulation of the United States, United Kingdom, Canada, India and the need for global harmonized practices. *Perspectives in Clinical Research* 9(4):170–174.

Harston, A. 2019. How the U.S. compares to Europe on biosimilar approvals and products in the pipeline. *Rothwell Figg*, October 29. https://www.biosimilarsip.com/2019/05/07/how-the-u-s-compares-to-europe-on-biosimilar-approvals-and-products-in-the-pipeline-4 (accessed September 13, 2019).

HC (Health Canada). 2018. *Australia Canada Singapore Switzerland (ACSS) Consortium–Erleada approval.* July 13. https://www.canada.ca/en/health-canada/corporate/transparency/regulatory-transparency-and-openness/improving-review-drugs-devices/notice-erleada.html (accessed September 24, 2019).

HSA (Health Sciences Authority). n.d. Update on ASEAN MRA on GMP conformity assessment for medicinal product registration in Singapore. https://www.hsa.gov.sg/content/dam/HSA/HPRG/Western_Medicine/Overview_Framework_Policies/Guidelines_on_Drug_Registration/Industry%20Updates/Update%20on%20ASEAN%20MRA%20GMP.pdf (accessed September 15, 2019).

Hunter, P. 2017. Advanced therapies push regulatory boundaries: Novel therapeutic approaches require more regulatory flexibility and transparency. *EMBO Reports* 18(12):2101–2104.

Hussaarts, L., S. Mühlebach, V. P. Shah, S. McNeil, G. Borchard, B. Flühmann, V. Weinstein, S. Neervannan, E. Griffiths, and W. Jiang. 2017. Equivalence of complex drug products: Advances in and challenges for current regulatory frameworks. *Annals of the New York Academy of Sciences* 1407(1):39–49.

IBEF (India Brand Equity Foundation). 2019. *Indian pharmaceuticals industry analysis.* https://www.ibef.org/industry/indian-pharmaceuticals-industry-analysis-presentation (accessed November 1, 2019).

ICH (International Council for Harmonisation of Technical Requirements for Pharmaceuticals for Human Use). 2016. *Integrated addendum to ICH E6(R1): Guideline for good clinical practice E6(R2).* https://www.ich.org/fileadmin/Public_Web_Site/ICH_Products/Guidelines/Efficacy/E6/E6_R2__Step_4_2016_1109.pdf (accessed September 17, 2019).

ICH. 2019. Welcome to the ICH official website. https://www.ich.org/home.html (accessed September 26, 2019).

ICMRA (International Coalition of Medicines Regulatory Authorities). 2017. *Capacity Building Working Group final report.* http://www.icmra.info/drupal/strategicinitiatives/capacitybuilding (accessed September 5, 2019).

ICMRA. 2019. International Coalition of Medicines Regulatory Authorities. http://www.icmra.info/drupal (accessed September 30, 2019).

ILAC (International Laboratory Accreditation Cooperation). 2019. ILAC's role. https://ilac.org/about-ilac/role (accessed September 10, 2019).

Indian Department of Pharmaceuticals. 2018. *Annual report 2017–2018.* https://pharmaceuticals.gov.in/sites/default/files/Annual%20Report%202017-18.pdf (accessed September 15, 2019).

IPRP (International Pharmaceutical Regulators Programme). 2019. International Pharmaceutical Regulators Programme. http://www.iprp.global/home (accessed September 28, 2019).

ISO (International Organization for Standardization). 2012. *ISO/IEC 17020:2012 conformity assessment—requirements for the operation of various types of bodies performing inspection*. https://www.iso.org/standard/52994.html (acccessed September 20, 2019).

Iyengar, S., L. Hedman, G. Forte, and S. Hill. 2016. Medicine shortages: A commentary on causes and mitigation strategies. *BMC Medicine* 14(1):124.

Kashoki, M., Z. Hanaizi, S. Yordanova, R. Veselý, C. Bouygues, J. Llinares, and S. L. Kweder. 2020. A comparison of EMA and FDA decisions for new drug marketing applications 2014–2016: Concordance, discordance, and why. *Clinical Pharmacology and Therapeutics* 107(1):195–202. doi: 10.1002/cpt.1565.

Khadem, A. 2019. WHO Regulatory Systems Strengthening Programme: WHO role in building effective and efficient regulatory systems for health products. World Health Organization. https://www.who.int/medicines/technical_briefing/tbs/TBS2019_WHO_RSS_Capacity_Building_GBT.pdf (accessed September 30, 2019).

Kulkarni, T. N., and N. G. Kulkarni. 2019. Authoring a periodic adverse drug experience report… here's what you need to know! *Perspectives in Clinical Research* 10(2):95–91.

La Entidad Mexicana de la Acreditación. 2019. International agreements. https://www.ema.org.mx/portal_v3/index.php/international-agreeementsi (accessed October 2, 2019).

Lesko, L. J., and J. Woodcock. 2004. Translation of pharmacogenomics and pharmacogenetics: a regulatory perspective. *Nature Reviews Drug Discovery* 3:763–769.

Luigetti, R., P. Bachmann, E. Cooke, and T. Salmonson. 2016. Collaboration, not competition: Developing new reliance models. *WHO Drug Information* 30(4):558–566.

Myles, P. S., E. Williamson, J. Oakley, and A. J. T. Forbes. 2014. Ethical and scientific considerations for patient enrollment into concurrent clinical trials. *Trials* 15(1):470.

Ni, J., J. Zhao, C. O. L. Ung, Y. Hu, H. Hu, and Y. J. G. Wang. 2017. Obstacles and opportunities in Chinese pharmaceutical innovation. *Globalization and Health* 13(Art. 21). doi: 10.1186/s12992-017-0244-6.

OECD (Organisation for Economic Co-operation and Development). 2013a. *International regulatory co-operation: Addressing global challenges*. Paris, France: OECD Publishing. doi: 10.1787/9789264200463-en.

OECD. 2013b. *OECD recommendation on the governance of clinical trials*. http://www.oecd.org/sti/inno/oecd-recommendation-governance-of-clinical-trials.pdf (accessed September 30, 2019).

OECD. 2014. *Regulatory enforcement and inspections*. https://www.oecd-ilibrary.org/content/publication/9789264208117-en (accessed September 27, 2019).

OECD. 2019. Good laboratory practice (GLP). https://www.oecd.org/chemicalsafety/testing/good-laboratory-practiceglp.htm (accessed September 27, 2019).

Office of the Director of National Intelligence. 2018. *Threats to pharmaceutical supply chains the public-private analytic exchange program research findings*. https://www.dni.gov/files/PE/Documents/2018_AEP-Pharmaceutical.pdf (accessed September 23, 2019).

PAHO (Pan American Health Organization). 2019a. PANDRH's members. https://www.paho.org/hq/index.php?option=com_content&view=article&id=11825:rede-parf-miembros&Itemid=41777&lang=en (accessed September 30, 2019).

PAHO. 2019b. *Regulatory reliance principles: Concept note and recommendations*. Ninth Conference of the Pan American Network for Drug Regulatory Harmonization (PANDRH) (San Salvador, October 24–26, 2018). http://iris.paho.org/xmlui/bitstream/handle/123456789/51549/PAHOHSS19003_eng.pdf (accessed September 16, 2019).

Paquette, M., J. Kelecevic, L. Schwartz, and R. Nieuwlaat. 2019. Ethical issues in competing clinical trials. *Contemporary Clinical Trials Communiations* 14:100352.

Patel, K., and N. Chotai. 2011. Documentation and records: Harmonized GMP requirements. *Journal of Young Pharmacists* 3(2):138–150.

Patel, P., N. McAuslane, and L. Liberti. 2019. *R&D briefing 71: Trends in the regulatory landscape for the approval of new medicines in Latin America*. London, UK: Centre for Innovation in Regulatory Science. http://www.cirsci.org/wp-content/uploads/2019/07/RD-briefing-71-Regulatory-trends-in-Latam-final-18719-cl.pdf (accessed September 29, 2019).

PIC/S (Pharmaceutical Inspection Co-operation Scheme). 2017. *Standard operating procedure: Procedure for handling rapid alerts and recalls arising from quality defects*. https://www.picscheme.org/layout/document.php?id=1140 (accessed September 3, 2019).

PIC/S. 2019a. Focused stakeholders consultation on revised draft PIC/S GMP guide annex 2a (manufacture of advanced therapy medicinal products for human use) and annex 2b (manufacture of biological medicinal substances and products for human use). News Release. https://picscheme.org/en/news?itemid=61 (accessed September 3, 2019).

PIC/S. 2019b. (Switzerland). Press release. PIC/S meetings in Geneva. https://picscheme.org/newsletters/5ce2547c0cf48 (accessed September 3, 2019).

PIC/S. 2019c. *Introduction*. https://picscheme.org/en/about-introduction (accessed September 30, 2019).

Ratanawijitrasin, S., and E. Wondemagegnehu. 2002. *Effective drug regulation: A multicountry study*. Geneva, Switzerland: WHO.

Ravinetto, R., H. Tinto, E. Diro, J. Okebe, Y. Mahendradhata, S. Rijal, E. Gotuzzo, P. Lutumba, A. Nahum, and K. J. B. De Nys. 2016. It is time to revise the international good clinical practices guidelines: Recommendations from non-commercial north–south collaborative trials. *BMJ Global Health* 1(3):e000122.

Rees, V. 2019a. The impact of counterfeit drugs in South and South-East Asia. *European Pharmaceutical Review*. https://www.europeanpharmaceuticalreview.com/article/92194/the-impact-of-counterfeit-drugs-in-south-and-south-east-asia (accessed September 30, 2019).

Rees, V. 2019b. US and India receive most warning letters from FDA. *European Pharmaceutical Review*. https://www.europeanpharmaceuticalreview.com/news/97201/us-and-india-receive-most-warning-letters-from-fda (accessed September 30, 2019).

Rönninger, S., S. Schmitt, V. Rangavajhula, E. Hough, and J. Lyda. 2012. Considerations on auditing and GXP requirements along the product lifecycle. *PDA Journal of Pharmaceutical Science and Technology* 66(5):396–402.

Roth, L., D. Bempong, J. B. Babigumira, S. Banoo, E. Cooke, D. Jeffreys, L. Kasonde, H. G. Leufkens, J. C. Lim, and M. J. G. Lumpkin. 2018. Expanding global access to essential medicines: Investment priorities for sustainably strengthening medical product regulatory systems. *Globalization and Health* 14(1):102.

Saint-Raymond, A. 2019. Mutual recognition agreements and reliance in the regulation of medicines. PowerPoint presentation at the July 10–11, 2019, meeting of the Committee on Mutual Recognition Agreements and Reliance in the Regulation of Medicines, London, UK.

Schwartz, M. 2017. Another brick in the wall: A new commitment implementing the mutual recognition of inspections. *FDA Law Blog*, August 24. http://www.fdalawblog.net/2017/08/another-brick-in-the-wall-a-new-commitment-implementing-the-mutual-recognition-of-inspections (accessed September 20, 2019).

Sravani, M., M. S. Kusuma, A. Prabhahar, and R. Nadendla. 2017. Registration of generic drugs in Central America and Mexico. *International Journal of Pharma and Chemical Research* 3(3):635–650.

TGA (Therapeutic Goods Administration). 2018. *Comparable overseas regulators (CORs) for prescription medicines: Criteria, COR report-based process and worksharing*. https://www.tga.gov.au/sites/default/files/comparable-overseas-regulators-cors-prescription-medicines.pdf (accessed October 20, 2019).

TGA. 2019a. ACSS–NAS work sharing initiative. https://www.tga.gov.au/acss-nas-work-sharing-initiative (accessed September 15, 2019).

TGA. 2019b. Australia–Canada–Singapore–Switzerland (ACSS) consortium. https://www.tga.gov.au/australia-canada-singapore-switzerland-acss-consortium (accessed September 15, 2019).

UNODC (United Nations Office on Drugs and Crime). 2019. *Transnational organized crime in Southeast Asia: Evolution, growth and impact.* https://www.unodc.org/documents/southeastasiaandpacific/Publications/2019/SEA_TOCTA_2019_web.pdf (accessed September 30, 2019).

VICH. 2019. What is VICH? https://www.vichsec.org/en/what-is-vich (accessed October 12, 2019).

Vinther, A. 2016. Drug shortage is a "wicked problem." *PDA Letter*, May 4. https://www.pda.org/pda-letter-portal/archives/full-article/drug-shortage-is-a-wicked-problem (accessed September 20, 2019).

WHO (World Health Organization). 2009. *Handbook: Good laboratory practice (GLP): Quality practices for regulated non-clinical research and development* (2nd ed.). https://www.who.int/tdr/publications/documents/glp-handbook.pdf (accessed September 5, 2019).

WHO. 2016a. Collaboration, not competition: Developing new reliance models. *WHO Drug Information* 30(4):558–566. https://www.who.int/medicines/publications/druginformation/WHO-DI_30-4_RegCollaboration.pdf (accessed September 21, 2019).

WHO. 2016b. *Good regulatory practices: Guidelines for national regulatory authorities for medical products.* https://www.who.int/medicines/areas/quality_safety/quality_assurance/GoodRegulatory_PracticesPublicConsult.pdf (accessed September 5, 2019).

WHO. 2016c. *WHO Zika virus research agenda.* https://www.who.int/reproductivehealth/zika/zika-virus-research-agenda/en (accessed September 22, 2019).

WHO. 2016d. Zika virus and complications: 2016 public health emergency of international concern. https://www.who.int/emergencies/zika-virus-tmp/en (accessed September 22, 2019).

WHO. 2017a. *China policies to promote local production of pharmaceutical products and protect public health.* https://www.who.int/phi/publications/2081China020517.pdf (accessed September 30, 2019).

WHO. 2017b. Prequalification process quality improvement initiatives: 2010–2016. *WHO Drug Information* 31(3):402–408.

WHO. 2018a. *Addressing the global shortage of, and access to, medicines and vaccines.* EB142/13. http://apps.who.int/gb/ebwha/pdf_files/EB142/B142_13-en.pdf (accessed September 30, 2019).

WHO. 2018b. *WHO Global Benchmarking Tool (GBT) for evaluation of national regulatory systems: Glossary and definitions.* https://www.who.int/medicines/regulation/10_GBT_Glossary_RevVI.pdf (accessed September 1, 2019).

WHO. 2019a. Essential medicines and health products: Pharmacovigilance. https://www.who.int/medicines/areas/quality_safety/safety_efficacy/pharmvigi/en (accessed September 24, 2019).

WHO. 2019b. Essential medicines and health products: Post market surveillance. https://www.who.int/medicines/regulation/ssffc/pms/en (accessed September 24, 2019).

WHO. 2019c. Essential medicines and health products: Prequalification of medicines—capacity building. https://extranet.who.int/prequal/content/capacity-building-0 (accessed September 24, 2019).

WHO. 2019d. Essential medicines and health products: Prequalification of medicines—WHO public inspection reports (WHOPRIS). https://extranet.who.int/prequal/key-resources/prequalification-reports/whopirs (accessed September 24, 2019).

WHO. 2019e. Essential medicines and health products: Why we need strong regulatory systems to reach universal health coverage. https://www.who.int/medicines/news/2019/strong-reg-systems-to-reach-UHC/en (accessed September 24, 2019).

WHO. 2019f. *Guidelines on the implementation of the WHO certification scheme on the quality of pharmaceutical products moving in international commerce*. https://www.who.int/medicines/areas/quality_safety/regulation_legislation/certification/guidelines/en/index2.html (accessed September 14, 2019).

WHO. 2019g. Immunization standards: National regulatory authorities. https://www.who.int/immunization_standards/national_regulatory_authorities/role/en (accessed September 24, 2019).

WHO. 2019h. International Conference of Drug Regulatory Authorities. https://www.who.int/medicines/areas/quality_safety/regulation_legislation/icdra/en (accessed September 14, 2019).

WHO. 2019i. WHO's approach to promoting reliance. Presentation at the 8th Asia Partnership Conference of Pharmaceutical Associations (APAC), 09 April 2019, Tokyo, Japan. https://apac-asia.com/images/achievements/pdf/8th/5_RA/09_WHO%E2%80%99s%20approach%20to%20promoting%20reliance.pdf (accessed September 24, 2019).

Wilkinson, E. 2019. India and China spark concerns for UK drug supplies. *Pharmaceutical Journal* 303(7928).

Wilson, B. J., and S. G. Nicholls. 2015. The Human Genome Project, and recent advances in personalized genomics. *Risk Management and Healthcare Policy* 8:9–20. doi: 10.2147/RMHP.S58728.

Zall Kusek, J., and R. Rist. 2004. *Ten steps to a results-based monitoring and evaluation system: A handbook for development practitioners*. https://www.oecd.org/dac/peer-reviews/World%20bank%202004%2010_Steps_to_a_Results_Based_ME_System.pdf (accessed September 12, 2019).

Zhai, M. Z., A. Sarpatwari, and A. S. Kesselheim. 2019. Why are biosimilars not living up to their promise in the US? *AMA Journal of Ethics* 21(8):E668–E678.

Appendix A

Glossary

Accountability: The result of the process which ensures that health actors take responsibility of what they are obliged to do and are made answerable for their actions.

Active pharmaceutical ingredient: Any substance or mixture of substances intended to be used in the manufacture of a drug (medicinal) product and that, when used in the production of a drug, becomes an active ingredient of the drug product. Such substances are intended to furnish pharmacological activity or other direct effect in the diagnosis, cure, mitigation, treatment, or prevention of disease or to affect the structure and function of the body.

Confidentiality commitment: A document that sets up the legal framework for a regulatory authority to share certain kinds of nonpublic information with regulatory counterparts in foreign countries and international organizations as part of cooperative law enforcement or regulatory activities.

Conformity assessment: A systematic examination to determine the extent to which a product, process, or service fulfills specified requirements.

Conformity assessment body: A body engaged in the performance of procedures for determining whether the relevant requirements in technical regulations or standards are fulfilled.

Effectiveness: The extent to which a specific intervention, procedure, regimen or service, when deployed in the field in routine circumstances, does what it is intended to do for a specified population.

Efficacy: The extent to which a specific intervention, procedure, regimen or service produces the intended result under ideal conditions.

Event: A specific identifiable happening or occurrence (e.g., the taking of a medicine; the experience of an adverse effect).

Falsified medical products: Medical products that deliberately/fraudulently misrepresent their identity, composition, or source.

Findings: See *Inspection observation.*

Good clinical practice (GCP): A standard for the design, conduct, performance, monitoring, auditing, recording, analysis, and reporting of clinical trials or studies. It provides assurance that the data and results that are reported are credible and accurate.

Good distribution practice (GDP): Describes the minimum standards that a wholesale distributor must meet to ensure that the quality and integrity of medicines is maintained throughout the supply chain.

Good manufacturing practice (GMP): The part of quality management that ensures that products are consistently produced and controlled to the quality standards appropriate to their intended use and as required by the marketing authorization, clinical trial authorization, or product specification.

Good pharmacovigilance practice (GPvP): Provides guidance for the appropriate oversight of products once they have been released onto the general market.

Inspection observation: A finding or statement of fact made during an inspection and substantiated by objective evidence. Such findings may be positive or negative. Positive observations should take the form of a description of the processes that the firm is carrying out particularly well and that may be considered as examples of particularly good practice. Negative observations are findings of noncompliance with requirements.

Medicinal products: In this report, a term that encompasses medicines and vaccines.

Monitoring: The continuous process of collecting and analyzing data to compare how well a project, program, or policy is being implemented against expected results.

Performance indicators: Measurable values used to quantify quality objectives to reflect the performance of an organization, process, or system, also known as "performance metrics" in some regions.

Post-marketing: The stage when a drug has been approved and is generally available on the market.

Promotion: All informational and persuasive activities by manufacturers and distributors, the intended effect of which is to induce the prescription, supply, purchase, and/or use of medicinal products.

Quality assurance: Is a wide-ranging concept covering all matters that individually or collectively influence the quality of a product. It is the totality of the arrangements made with the object of ensuring that pharmaceutical products are of the quality required for their intended use. With regard to pharmaceuticals, quality assurance can be divided into major areas: development, quality control, production, distribution, and inspections.

Recognition: The routine acceptance by the regulatory authority (RA) in one jurisdiction of the work products and regulatory decisions of another RA or other trusted institution.

Regulatory authority: See *Regulatory system*.

Regulatory framework: The collection of laws, regulations, guidelines, and other regulatory instruments through which a government controls the manufacture, clinical evaluation, marketing, promotion, and post-marketing safety benchmarking of medical products.

Regulatory system: The system composed of entities responsible for the registration, marketing authorization, and other regulatory functions concerning medical products. The number of regulatory entities responsible for different regulatory functions may vary from one country to another (i.e., the regulatory authority may or may not be a single entity). The terms *national medicines regulatory authority* (NMRA) and/or *drug regulatory authority* (DRA) are also used, although less encouraged, to designate the national regulatory authority.

Reliance: The act whereby the regulatory authority in one jurisdiction may take into account and give significant weight to (i.e., totally or partially rely on work products by another regulatory authority or trusted institution in reaching its own decision). The relying authority remains responsible and accountable for decisions taken, even when it relies on the decisions and information of others.

Substandard and falsified medicines: Authorized medicines that fail to meet either their quality standards or their specifications, or both.

Substandard medicines (also called "out of specification"): Authorized medicines that fail to meet either their quality standards or their specifications, or both.

Unilateral reliance: A lower-resourced authority that bases its decision on the work product of a well-resourced authority.

Work sharing: The act whereby two or more medicines regulatory agencies agree to work together on a specific regulatory activity. Such work sharing may be on a reactive ad hoc basis or an established proactive routine basis. Such work sharing may result in a common decision.

Appendix B

Table of Mutual Recognition Agreements

Mutual Recognition Agreements (MRAs) in the Regulation of Medicines

Country	Partners	Operational Date	Process	Products
Australia	Canada	January 1, 2006	GMP inspections and batch certification	Therapeutic goods, including active pharmaceutical ingredients.
	European Economic Area (Iceland, Norway, Liechtenstein)	July 1, 2000	GMP inspections and batch certification	The definition of medicinal products includes all human and veterinary products, such as chemical and biological pharmaceuticals; immunologicals; radiopharmaceuticals; stable medicinal products derived from human blood or human plasma; premixes for the preparation of veterinary medicated feedstuffs; and, where appropriate, vitamins, minerals, herbal remedies, and homeopathic medicinal products.
	European Union (EU)	January 1, 1999; June 2001 for veterinary medicines	GMP inspections and batch certification	Human chemical pharmaceuticals; medicinal gases; human biologicals, including vaccines, immunologicals, and biotherapeutics; human radiopharmaceuticals; stable medicinal products derived from human blood or human plasma; homeopathic medicines, if classified as medicinal products; vitamins, minerals, and herbal medicines if classified as medicinal products; products intended for use in clinical trials, investigational medicinal products, except those used in phase I clinical trials; intermediate products and bulk pharmaceuticals; active pharmaceutical ingredients, only for human medicinal products; veterinary chemical pharmaceuticals; premixes for the preparation of veterinary medicated feedstuffs; veterinary immunologicals, including vaccines, immunologicals, and biotherapeutics.
	New Zealand	January 1, 1997	Product standards, manufacturing standards; conformance assessment requirements, packaging and labeling standards	Therapeutic goods

	Singapore	July 1, 2001	GMP inspections and batch certification	Medicinal products
Canada	European Economic Area (Iceland, Norway, Liechtenstein)	November 2002	GMP inspections and batch certification	Human pharmaceuticals including prescription and non-prescription drugs and medicinal gases; human biologicals including vaccines, stable medicinal products derived from human blood or human plasma, biotherapeutics, and immunologicals; human radiopharmaceuticals; veterinary pharmaceuticals, including prescription and nonprescription drugs, and premixes for the preparation of veterinary medicated feedstuffs; where appropriate, vitamins, minerals, herbal remedies, and homeopathic medicinal products; active pharmaceutical ingredients or bulk pharmaceuticals. (Note: Active pharmaceutical ingredients are not GMP regulated.) Clarifications: Manufactured drugs used in clinical trials (Note: Currently limited to sites already holding a manufacturing authorization/establishment license); natural health products (NHPs) (Note: Currently, certificates of compliance are provided by MRA partners. In Canada, regulatory amendments are being prepared that will allow Canadian NHP companies to hold an establishment license in addition to the site license required under the NHP regulations); and human biologicals. (Note: The MRA covers GMP evidence for manufacturing sites of human biologicals. It does not address the Canadian requirements for lot-to-lot release of these products as set forth under Section C.04.015 of the Food and Drug Regulations.) Temporary exclusions: Stable medicinal products derived from human blood or human plasma; active pharmaceutical ingredients or bulk pharmaceuticals. Definite exclusions: Blood and blood components; veterinary biologics.

continued

Mutual Recognition Agreements (MRAs) in the Regulation of Medicines				
Country	Partners	Operational Date	Process	Products
	EU	February 2003	GMP inspections and batch certification	Human pharmaceuticals including prescription and non-prescription drugs and medicinal gases; human biologicals including vaccines, stable medicinal products derived from human blood or human plasma, biotherapeutics, and immunologicals; human radiopharmaceuticals; veterinary pharmaceuticals, including prescription and nonprescription drugs, and premixes for the preparation of veterinary medicated feedstuffs; where appropriate, vitamins, minerals, herbal remedies, and homeopathic medicinal products; active pharmaceutical ingredients or bulk pharmaceuticals. (Note: Active pharmaceutical ingredients are not GMP regulated.) Clarifications: Manufactured drugs used in clinical trials (Note: Currently limited to sites already holding a manufacturing authorization/establishment license); NHPs (Note: Currently, certificates of compliance are provided by MRA partners. In Canada, regulatory amendments are being prepared that will allow Canadian NHP companies to hold an establishment license in addition to the site license required under the NHP regulations); pre-authorization/pre-marketing GMP inspections (Note: As of October 1, 2004, the pre-authorization/pre-marketing GMP inspections are included within the scope of the MRA); human biologicals. (Note: The MRA covers GMP evidence for manufacturing sites of human biologicals. It does not address the Canadian requirements for lot-to-lot release of these products as set forth under Section C.04.015 of the Food and Drug Regulations.)

				Temporary exclusions: Stable medicinal products derived from human blood or human plasma; active pharmaceutical ingredients or bulk pharmaceuticals. Definite exclusions: Blood and blood components; veterinary biologics.

continued

Mutual Recognition Agreements (MRAs) in the Regulation of Medicines				
Country	Partners	Operational Date	Process	Products
	Switzerland	June 2000	GMP inspections, GLP, and batch certification	Human pharmaceuticals including prescription and non-prescription drugs and medicinal gases; human biologicals including vaccines, stable medicinal products derived from human blood or human plasma, biotherapeutics, and immunologicals; human radiopharmaceuticals; veterinary pharmaceuticals, including prescription and nonprescription drugs and premixes for the preparation of veterinary medicated feedstuffs; where appropriate, vitamins, minerals, herbal remedies, and homeopathic medicinal products; active pharmaceutical ingredients or bulk pharmaceuticals. (Note: Active pharmaceutical ingredients are not GMP regulated.) Clarifications: Manufactured drugs used in clinical trials (Note: Currently limited to sites already holding a manufacturing authorization/establishment license); NHPs (Note: Currently, certificates of compliance are provided by MRA partners. In Canada, regulatory amendments are being prepared that will allow Canadian NHP companies to hold an establishment license in addition to the site license required under the NHP regulations); human biologicals. (Note: The MRA covers GMP evidence for manufacturing sites of human biologicals. It does not address the Canadian requirements for lot-to-lot release of these products as set forth under Section C.04.015 of the Food and Drug Regulations.) Temporary exclusions: Stable medicinal products derived from human blood or human plasma; active pharmaceutical ingredients or bulk pharmaceuticals.

				Definite exclusions: Blood and blood components; and veterinary biologics.
EEA	Switzerland	June 1, 2002	GMP inspections, GLP, and batch certification	The definition of drugs encompasses all products for human and veterinary use, including chemical and biological pharmaceutical, immunological, and radiopharmaceutical products; stable drugs derived from blood and human plasma; premixes for the manufacture of medicated feed; and, where appropriate, vitamins, minerals, medicinal herbs, and homeopathic medicines.
EU	Israel*	January 2013	The MRA with Israel is an agreement on conformity assessment and acceptance of industrial products	Human chemical and biological pharmaceuticals; human immunologicals; radiopharmaceuticals; vitamins, minerals, and herbal medicines if classified as medicinal products; intermediate products and bulk pharmaceuticals; active pharmaceutical ingredients; excipients; veterinary chemical pharmaceuticals; premixes and preparation of veterinary medicated feedstuffs; veterinary biologicals except immunologicals. Israel and the EU recognize official batch releases carried out by each other's authorities.
	Japan	May 29, 2004, with limited scope, updated scope July 2018	GMP inspections, GLP, and batch certification	Original scope (subsequently amended in 2018): human medicines only, including chemical pharmaceuticals; homeopathic medicinal products if classified as medicinal products and subject to GMP requirements in Japan; vitamins, minerals, and herbal medicines if classified as medicines by both parties; biological pharmaceuticals, including immunologicals and vaccines, that are produced by cell culture utilizing natural or recombinant microorganisms or established cell lines or derived from nontransgenic plants and nontransgenic animals; active pharmaceutical ingredients of any medicine covered in the agreement; sterile medicines that belong to any of the above categories.

continued

Mutual Recognition Agreements (MRAs) in the Regulation of Medicines

Country	Partners	Operational Date	Process	Products
	New Zealand	January 1, 1999, for human medicines; June 1, 2001, for veterinary medicines	GMP inspections and batch certification	Human chemical pharmaceuticals; medicinal gases; human biologicals, including vaccines, immunologicals, and biotherapeutics; human radiopharmaceuticals; stable medicinal products derived from human blood or human plasma; homeopathic medicines if classified as medicinal products; vitamins, minerals, and herbal medicines if classified as medicinal products; products intended for use in clinical trials; IMPs; intermediate products and bulk pharmaceuticals; veterinary chemical pharmaceuticals; premixes for preparation of veterinary medicated feedstuffs; veterinary immunologicals, including vaccines, immunologicals, and biotherapeutics.
	Switzerland	June 2002	GMP inspections, GLP, and batch certification	Human chemical pharmaceuticals; medicinal gases; human biologicals, including vaccines, immunologicals, and biotherapeutics; human radiopharmaceuticals; stable medicinal products derived from human blood or human plasma; advanced-therapy medicinal products; homeopathic medicines if classified as medicinal products; vitamins, minerals, and herbal medicines if classified as medicinal products; products intended for use in clinical trials (IMPs); active pharmaceutical ingredients; intermediate products and bulk pharmaceuticals; veterinary chemical pharmaceuticals; premixes for preparation of veterinary medicated feedstuffs; veterinary immunologicals, including vaccines, immunologicals, and biotherapeutics. Switzerland and the EU recognize official batch releases carried out by each other's authorities.

	United States	Entered into force on December 1, 1998, but was in transition phase until July 2019	GMP inspections and batch certification	Human chemical pharmaceuticals; medicinal gases; human biologicals, including immunologicals and biotherapeutics; human radiopharmaceuticals; homeopathic medicines if classified as medicinal products; vitamins, minerals, and herbal medicines if classified as medicinal products; active pharmaceutical ingredients; intermediate products and bulk pharmaceuticals. Acceptance of batch testing certificates postponed until the U.S. Food and Drug Administration recognizes all EU Member States.

NOTES: EEA = European Economic Area; EU = European Union; GLP = good laboratory practice; GMP = good manufacturing practice; IMP = investigational medicinal product; NHP = natural health product.

*"Israel adopted the relevant legislation amendments in the field of pharmaceuticals, which ensured the application of European GMP requirements" (Aronov et al., 2019, p. 594).

Appendix C

Table of Global Good Manufacturing Practice (GMP) Reliance Initiatives Based on the International Coalition of Medicines Regulatory Authorities' Mapping Exercise

Initiative	Objective	Scope	
I. Single Unified System			
European Union (EU) Inspection System	A single European GMP inspection system	GMP inspections of the manufacturers of active pharmaceutical ingredients (APIs) and finished dosage forms	
II. Reliance-Focused			
Mutual recognition agreement (MRA)	Legally binding treaty between two participating parties and exchange of GMP certificates based on equivalent GMP compliance program	May cover human and veterinary products	
Association of Southeast Asian Nations (ASEAN) MRA	Recognition of GMP inspection of manufacturers of medicinal products among 10 ASEAN Member States	Medicinal products in finished dosage forms; excludes such products as biopharmaceuticals, radiopharmaceuticals, traditional medicines, and investigational medicinal products	
European Medicines Agency (EMA)/U.S. Food and Drug Administration (FDA)/ Therapeutic Goods Administration (TGA) API program	To foster cooperation and mutual confidence among participating regulators through better communication and exchange of information on inspection planning	Joint inspections of API manufacturers located outside the participating regions; reliance on API inspections by other authorities; extended inspections on behalf of other countries	
EMA/FDA mutual reliance confidence building*	Allows some inspections on each other's territories to be deferred or waived completely based on a number of considerations	The strategy is applicable to GMP inspections related to manufacturing sites located in the United States and the European Economic Area involving products for both human and veterinary use	

	Membership	Frequency of Meetings	Work Products
	Austria, Belgium, Bulgaria, Croatia, Cyprus, the Czech Republic, Denmark, Estonia, Finland, France, Germany, Greece, Hungary, Iceland, Ireland, Italy, Latvia, Liechtenstein, Lithuania, Luxembourg, Malta, the Netherlands, Norway, Poland, Portugal, Romania, Slovakia, Slovenia, Spain, Sweden, United Kingdom	Multiple meetings	1. (non-exhaustive) Reliance on GMP inspections performed by any EU authority, common inspection procedures, common approach to training and qualifications of inspectors 2. Rapid alert system for quality defects 3. Joint Audit Program
	Bilateral between individual countries and/or regions	Ongoing teleconferences as the confidence-building phase is evolving	1. Ongoing communication (e.g., Joint Sectoral Group meetings, exchange of annual maintenance reports, ad hoc MRA partners meeting) 2. Similar, not identical approaches
	Brunei, Cambodia, Indonesia, Laos, Malaysia, Burma (Myanmar), the Philippines, Singapore, Thailand, Vietnam	Not applicable	Under this MRA, all ASEAN Member States shall accept and recognize the GMP certificates and/or inspection reports of a listed inspection service
	Australian Therapeutic Goods Administration (TGA), European Directorate of the Quality of Medicines and HealthCare (EDQM), European Medicines Agency (EMA), European National Supervisory Authorities, U.S. Food and Drug Administration (FDA), World Health Organization (WHO)	Monthly teleconferences	1. Joint inspections 2. Reliance on inspections by other authorities 3. Feedback
	Not applicable	Ad hoc meetings	Under this MRA, all EU Member States shall accept and recognize the GMP certificates and/or inspection reports, and batch testing reports of the United States and vice versa

continued

Initiative	Objective	Scope	
EU API listing	Listing of a country as having GMP inspection and supervision standards equivalent to those in the EU	APIs only	
III. Cooperation-Focused			
Pan American Health Organization (PAHO)/WHO Latin American Initiative	1. Establishment of cooperation mechanisms that will make it possible to strengthen the steering role for other national regulatory authorities 2. Cooperation actions for GMP are being conducted to strengthen capacity building of Central American and Caribbean regulatory authorities	Some technical cooperation on marketing authorization and inspections International inspections Periodic audits of NRA	
EMA/FDA Finished Products program*	The overall objective is to see whether greater international collaboration can help to better distribute inspection capacity, allowing more sites to be monitored and reducing unnecessary duplication		

Membership	Frequency of Meetings	Work Products
Bilateral between EU and country requesting list	Not applicable	Country listed as equivalent
Steering committee: Argentina, Brazil, Colombia, Cuba, Mexico	Two meetings annually (one at PAHO/ Washington and the other at one of the Steering Committee countries)	1. Audits of national regulatory capabilities 2. Cooperation mechanisms for inspections 3. Recognition of regulatory capacity in inspections
EMA, FDA	Initially monthly meetings, then ad hoc	Joint inspections

continued

Initiative	Objective	Scope	
Pharmaceutical Inspection Co-operation Scheme (PIC/S)	1. International cooperation in the area of GMP 2. Developing and promoting harmonized GMP standards and guidance documents 3. Training GMP inspectors 4. Assessing (and reassessing) GMP inspectorates 5. Facilitating cooperation and networking and planning of inspection	Initially restricted to medicinal products for human use; now some veterinary authorities are included Initially restricted to finished products; currently being extended to APIs Good distribution practice (GDP) added to mandate New Expert Circle on PIC/S good clinical practice (GCP) and good pharmacovigilance practice (GPvP)	

Membership	Frequency of Meetings	Work Products
Argentinian National Institute of Drugs (INAME), Australian Therapeutic Goods Administration (TGA), Austrian Medicines and Medical Devices Agency (AGES), Belgian Federal Agency for Medicines and Health Products (AFMPS-FAGG), Canadian Health Products and Food Branch Inspectorate (HPFBI)—Health Canada, Agency for Medicinal Products and Medical Devices of Croatia (HALMED), Cypriot Pharmaceutical Services (CyPHS), Czech State Institute for Drug Control (SÚKL), Czech Institute for State Control of Veterinary Biologicals and Medicines (ISCVBM), Danish Health and Medicines Authority (DKMA), Estonian State Agency of Medicines (SAM), Finnish Medicines Agency (FIMEA), French National Agency for Medicines and Health Products Safety (ANSM), French Agency for Food, Environmental & Occupational Health Safety (ANSES), German Federal Ministry of Health (BMG), Central Authority of the Laender for Health Protection regarding Medicinal Products and Medical Devices (ZLG) (BMG and ZLG count as one PIC/S Participating Authority), Greek National Organisation for Medicines (EOF), Pharmacy and Poisons Board of Hong Kong (PPBHK), Hungarian National Institute of Pharmacy and Nutrition (NIPN), Icelandic Medicines Agency (IMA), Indonesian National Agency for Drug and Food Control (NADFC), Iran Food and Drug Administration (IFDA), Irish Health Products Regulatory Authority (HPRA), Israeli Institute for Standardization and Control of Pharmaceuticals (ISCP), Italian Medicines Agency (AIFA), Japanese Ministry of Health, Labour and Welfare (MHLW), Japanese Pharmaceuticals and Medical Devices (*continues*)	Twice per year for the Committee of Officials Once per year for seminar and experts circles	1. Training activities/ seminars/dexpert circles 2. Guidance documents for inspectorates and industry 3. Harmonized inspections procedure 4. Reports on audited inspectorates

continued

Initiative	Objective	Scope	

Membership	Frequency of Meetings	Work Products
Agency (PMDA) (MHLW and PMDA count as one PIC/S Participating Authority), Korea (Republic of) Ministry of Food and Drug Safety (MFDS), Latvian State Agency of Medicine (ZVA), Liechtenstein's Office of Healthcare (AG), Lithuanian State Medicines Control Agency (SMCA), Malaysian National Pharmaceutical Regulatory Agency (NPRA), Maltese Medicines Authority (MAM), Mexican Federal Commission for the Protection Against Sanitary Risks (COFEPRIS), Dutch Health Care Inspectorate (IGZ), New Zealand's Medicines and Medical Devices Safety Authority (Medsafe), Norwegian Medicines Agency (NOMA), Polish Chief Pharmaceutical Inspectorate (CPI), Portuguese National Authority of Medicines and Health Products, IP (INFARMED IP), Romanian National Agency for Medicines and Medical Devices (NAMMD), Singapore's Health Sciences Authority (HSA), Slovak State Institute for Drug Control (SIDC), Slovenian Agency for Medicinal Products and Medical Devices (JAZMP), South African Health Products Regulatory Authority (SAHPRA), Spanish Agency of Medicines and Medical Devices (AEMPS) (The competence for GMP/GDP inspections in Spain is shared between the central authority, Spanish Agency for Medicines and Medical Devices [AEMPS], and the Spanish regional authorities, which count as one PIC/S Participating Authority. All Spanish Medicinal Authorities, which are listed on the AEMPS web site, are considered as PIC/S Participating Authorities and are represented in PIC/S by the AEMPS), Swedish Medical Products Agency (MPA), Swiss Agency for Therapeutic Products (Swissmedic), Taiwan Food and Drug Administration (TFDA), (*continues*)		

continued

Initiative	Objective	Scope	

NOTES: The original table includes the following disclaimer: "The information on this table has been compiled by EMA according to the available information. As in certain cases it is difficult to have accurate or up-to-date information and there are continuous changes, EMA strongly recommends to check the information with the relevant websites or directly with the relevant organizations."

*These initiatives are closely related. EMA/FDA mutual reliance confidence building derived from EMA/FA Finished Products Program.

SOURCE: Adapted from EMA, 2016.

	Membership	Frequency of Meetings	Work Products
	Thai Food and Drug Administration (Thai FDA), Turkish Medicines and Medical Devices Agency (TMMDA), State Service of Ukraine on Medicines and Drugs Control (SMDC), United Kingdom's Medicines & Healthcare products Regulatory Agency (MHRA), United Kingdom's Veterinary Medicine Directorate (VMD), U.S. Food and Drug Administration (FDA) Partner to PIC/S: European Directorate for the Quality of Medicines and HealthCare, EMA-European medicines		

Appendix D

Study Methods

The U.S. Food and Drug Administration's (FDA's) Office of International Programs (now the Office of Global Policy and Strategy) commissioned the National Academies of Sciences, Engineering, and Medicine to review and assess the current and potential use of mutual recognition agreements (MRAs) and other reliance-based procedures in the regulation of medicines. The National Academies assembled an expert committee to examine the ways these tools are being used, as well as the benefits, risks, and challenges associated with such arrangements.

LITERATURE SEARCH

An extensive search of the literature was conducted. The search parameters included publications after 2005 in English, Spanish, and French drawn from peer-reviewed journals, law reviews, and the grey literature. Databases searched included Embase, Lexis Law Reviews, Medline, PubMed, and Scopus. Organizational reviews were also conducted to include the Organisation for Economic Co-operation and Development (OECD), the World Trade Organization, and the World Health Organization. Primary search terms were Mutual Recognition Agreements, MRA, and Reliance. There were 40 secondary search terms grouped into four areas: functions, implementation, authorities, and individual nations. This search returned 110 articles.

ONLINE SEARCHES

For the landscaping, more recent information not contained in the standard searches was required. Therefore, the literature search was supplemented with online searches that consisted mainly of searching governmental websites for documents and other reports.

MEETINGS AND INFORMATION-GATHERING SESSIONS

During the course of the year-long study, the committee held four in-person meetings (February, April, July, and September 2019). The April and July committee meetings included portions open to the public; the agendas for those open sessions appear below. In addition to the committee meetings, 14 information-gathering sessions were held with key parties through virtual teleconferences and in-person meetings.

Open meetings and information-gathering sessions were organized to facilitate direct conversation between committee members and the regulators of various countries. The overall objectives of the open meetings and information-gathering sessions were to gather input from a wide range of interested parties on their experience with and use of mutual recognition/reliance agreements and informal practices of recognition/reliance, which allow regulators to use information from their counterparts at foreign drug regulatory agencies, in medicines regulation.

All of the information-gathering sessions observed the same general format beginning with opening remarks from the committee chair, followed by remarks from the participant(s) based on guiding questions, and concluding with a discussion between the participant(s) and committee members. Given the varying international locations of the experts, most of these sessions were held through virtual teleconference software. The dates and participants for each information-gathering session are provided below.

ADDITIONAL FEEDBACK

As part of the fact-finding process, the committee and project staff compiled and distributed to the regulatory authorities of various countries a committee-developed supplemental information-gathering questionnaire consisting of four questions regarding information sharing, work sharing, recognition of other agencies' decisions, and recognition of regulatory standards. Depending on the answers given to these questions, supplemental questions were posed to help the committee better understand the landscape of MRAs and other reliance-based procedures in the regulation of medicines. The committee and project staff received and utilized four sets of responses to supplement their other methods of information gathering.

PUBLIC COMMITTEE MEETING AGENDAS

Open Meeting 1:
Date: April 1, 2019
Location: National Academy of Sciences
2101 Constitution Avenue, NW, Washington, DC 20418

OPEN SESSION 1

9:25 am **OPENING REMARKS**
Alastair Wood, Committee Chair

9:30 am **MUTUAL RECOGNITION AND PUBLIC HEALTH: POTENTIAL BENEFITS AND CHALLENGES**
Moderator: Alastair Wood

Jonathan "Jono" Quick
Former Director, Essential Medicines and Pharmaceutical Policies, World Health Organization, and Senior Fellow Emeritus, Management Sciences for Health (virtual connection)

10:00 am **THE VALUE OF MRAs: LEVERAGING EFFICIENCIES FOR GREATER PUBLIC HEALTH PROTECTION**
Dara Corrigan
Fresenius Kabi/formerly with U.S. Food and Drug Administration

11:00 am Break—Adjourn open session

11:15 am **DEBRIEF**

12:00 pm **WORKING LUNCH: PREPARE FOR OPEN SESSION 2**
Lunch available in cafeteria, please return to meeting room for closed session discussion

1:00 pm **EXPLORE GOALS AND QUESTIONS FOR OPEN SESSION 2**

OPEN SESSION 2

1:30 pm **RECONVENE**
Alastair Wood, Committee Chair

1:35 pm **CURRENT MRA PERSPECTIVES FROM FDA**
Mary Ann Slack, U.S. Food and Drug Administration

2:20 pm **FINANCIAL EFFICIENCES DERIVED FROM MEXICO'S MRAs**
Julio Sánchez y Tépoz
ALó ProSciences/formerly with Federal Commission for the Protection against Sanitary Risks, Mexico

3:00 pm **THREE EXAMPLES OF MUTUAL RECOGNITION FROM THE BRAZILIAN PERSPECTIVE**
Dirceu Barbano
Former Director-Chairman, Brazilian Health Regulatory Agency (virtual connection)

3:30 pm Adjourn open session

Open Meeting 2:
Date: July 10, 2019
Location: Bill & Melinda Gates Foundation—London Office
62 Buckingham Gate, London SW1E 6AJ

8:30 am **WELCOME**
Mary Lou Valdez
Associate Commissioner for Diplomacy and Partnership
Office of Global Policy and Strategy
U.S. Food and Drug Administration

8:35 am **OPENING REMARKS**
Alastair Wood, Committee Chair

9:00 am **SESSION I: INFORMATION EXCHANGE AND USE AND SCOPE OF EXCHANGED INFORMATION PRESENTATIONS WITH FACILIATATED DISCUSSIONS**
National Regulatory Agencies 10-minute remarks, followed by facilitated discussion

REGULATORS—PART 1

9:00 am **Alison Cossar (virtual)**
Manager, Pre-Market Medicine Group
Medsafe, Ministry of Health, New Zealand

Kaylene Raynes and Adrian Bootes (virtual)
Kaylene Raynes
Director, Applications & Advisory Management
Prescription Medicines Authorisation Branch, Therapeutic Goods Administration, Australia

Adrian Bootes
Branch head, Prescription Medicines Authorisation
Therapeutic Goods Administration, Australia

Jörg Schläpfer and Federico Cimini
Jörg Schläpfer
Sector Management Services and International Affairs
Swiss Agency for Therapeutic Products (Swissmedic)

Federico Cimini
Head of Division Inspectorates
Swiss Agency for Therapeutic Products (Swissmedic)

9:30 am **Group Discussion**

10:00 am **BREAK**

REGULATORS—PART 2

10:20 am **Siu Ping Lam**
Director, Licensing Division
Medicines & Healthcare products Regulatory Agency, United Kingdom

Agnes Saint-Raymond and Brendan Cuddy
Agnes Saint-Raymond
Head of International Affairs Division
European Medicines Agency

Brendan Cuddy
Head of Manufacturing Quality and Supply Chain Integrity
European Medicines Agency

Dominique De Backer
Policy Officer, Pharmaceutical Unit at DG Health and Food Safety
European Commission

John Lynch
GMP Inspector and Senior Inspector
Health Products Regulatory Authority, Ireland

11:00 am **Group Discussion**

12:30 pm **LUNCH**

SESSION II: STAKEHOLDER INPUT
Input from stakeholder, 15-minute remarks, followed by facilitated discussion

1:30 pm **International Organization (virtual)**
Emer Cooke
Director, Regulation of Medicines and Other Health Technologies
World Health Organization

Facilitated discussion and questions from the committee

2:30 pm **Industry**
Janis Bernat and Rebecca Lumsden

Janis Bernat
Director, Biotherapeutics and Scientific Affairs
International Federation of Pharmaceutical Manufacturers & Associations

Rebecca Lumsden
Director–EM Regulatory Policy, Pfizer
On behalf of International Federation of Pharmaceutical Manufacturers & Associations

Facilitated discussion and questions from the committee

3:15 pm **Patient Group**
Kawaldip Sehmi
Chief Executive Officer
International Alliance of Patients' Organizations

Facilitated discussion and questions from the committee

4:00 pm Adjourn open session

Information-Gathering Sessions

Meeting 1 (Virtual):

Date: May 3, 2019
Country/regulatory agency: United Kingdom, Medicines & Healthcare products Regulatory Agency
Participant(s): Ian Hudson, Chief Executive

Meeting 2 (Virtual):

Date: May 7, 2019
Country/regulatory agency: European Union, European Medicines Agency
Participant(s): Agnes Saint-Raymond, Head of International Affairs Division, Head of Portfolio Board; Tania Teixeira, European Medicines Agency Liaison Official, U.S. Food and Drug Administration

Meeting 3 (Virtual):

Date: May 28, 2019
Country/regulatory agency: Switzerland, Swissmedic
Participant(s): Petra Doerr, Head of Sector Communication and Networking; other Swissmedic staff members; Raimund T. Bruhin, Executive Director

Meeting 4 (Virtual):

Date: May 29, 2019
Country/regulatory agency: Spain, Agencia Española de Medicamentos y Productos Sanitarios (Spain's Agency for Medicines and Health Products)
Participant(s): Belén Escribano, Head of Pharmaceutical Inspection and Enforcement Department; Manuel Ibarra Lorente, Head, Area of Inspection of Standards of GMP and GLP; R. San José Rodriguez, Department of Inspection and Control of Medicines; Jesús Díaz Hernández, Technical Advisor, Quality Unit and Secretariat Technical Inspection Committee, Department of Drug Inspection and Control

Meeting 5 (Virtual):

Date: May 31, 2019
Country/regulatory agency: Canada, Health Canada
Participant(s): Kimby Barton, Director, Health Products Inspection & Licensing (HPIL); Linsey Hollett, Acting Director General, Health Product Compliance Directorate (HPCD); Stephen McCaul, GMP Manager; Stéphanie Anctil, MRA Officer

(HPIL); Louise Kane, Manager, MRA and International Affairs Program; Celina Bak, Acting Associate Director, Health Product Compliance and Risk Management (HPCRM); Ann Kourtesis, Acting GMP Manager–Foreign Sites; Joy Bregg, Acting GMP Manager–Domestic; Kim Dayman-Rutkus, Senior Policy Advisor, Policy and Regulatory Strategies Directorate

Meeting 6 (Virtual):

Date: June 6, 2019
Country/regulatory agency: Pharmaceutical Inspection Convention and the Pharmaceutical Inspection Co-operation Scheme
Participant(s): Anne Hayes, Deputy Chair; John Lynch, former member of the Committee of Officials of Pharmaceutical Inspection Co-operation Scheme

Meeting 7 (Virtual):

Date: June 10, 2019
Country/regulatory agency: United States, Food and Drug Administration
Participant(s): Peter Marks, Director of the Center for Biologics Evaluation and Research

Meeting 8 (Virtual):

Date: June 10, 2019
Country/regulatory agency: United States, Food and Drug Administration
Participant(s): Janet Woodcock, Director of the Center for Drug Evaluation and Research

Meeting 9 (Virtual):

Date: June 10, 2019
Country/regulatory agency: Australia, Therapeutic Goods Administration
Participant(s): Kaylene Raynes, Director, Applications & Advisory Management; Jane Cook, First Assistant Secretary, Medicines Regulation Division, Prescription Medicines Authorisation; Adrian Bootes, Branch Head, Prescription Medicines Authorisation; Tracey Duffy, First Assistant Secretary, Medical Devices and Product Quality Division; Joe Hlubucek, Senior Policy Officer, International Regulatory Coordination Section

Meeting 10 (In-person):
Date: June 11, 2019
Country/regulatory agency: United States, Food and Drug Administration
Participant(s): Mark Abdoo, Associate Commissioner of the Office of Global Policy and Strategy

Meeting 11 (Virtual):
Date: June 26, 2019
Country/regulatory agency: International Generic and Biosimilar Medicines Association
Participant(s): Suzette Kox, Secretary General

Meeting 12 (Virtual):
Date: July 24, 2019
Country/regulatory agency: Singapore, Health Sciences Authority
Participant(s): Chan Chen Leng, Group Director, Health Products Regulation Group (HPRG); Jessica Teo, Division Director, Audit and Licensing Branch, HPRG; Agnes Chan, Director, Therapeutic Products Branch, HPRG; Chua Siew Wei, Deputy Director, Stakeholder Engagement Office, HPRG

Meeting 13 (In-person):
Date: July 29, 2019
Country/regulatory association: United States, Association for Accessible Medicines
Participant(s): David R. Gaugh, Senior Vice President for Sciences and Regulatory Affairs; Lisa Parks, Vice President for Sciences and Regulatory Affairs

Meeting 14 (Virtual):
Date: August 2, 2019
Country/regulatory agency: Medicines & Healthcare products Regulatory Agency
Participant(s): Jonathan Mogford, Director of Policy

Appendix E

Committee Member Biographies

Alastair J. J. Wood, MB, ChB, FRCP, FACP (NAM) (*Chair*), was professor of both medicine and pharmacology at Vanderbilt University Medical School and served as assistant vice chancellor for clinical research and associate dean, Vanderbilt Medical School, before being appointed emeritus professor of medicine and emeritus professor of pharmacology in 2006. He was a partner at Symphony Capital LLC, a private equity company investing in the clinical development of novel biopharmaceutical products, from 2006 to 2018. He has also periodically consulted for pharmaceutical companies (AMAG, Sanofi, etc.) in the past 12 months. Dr. Wood has been honored by being elected to the National Academy of Medicine, the American Association of Physicians, and the American Society for Clinical Investigation; is an honorary fellow of the American Gynecological and Obstetrical Society; and was awarded fellowships of the American College of Physicians, the Royal College of Physicians of London, and the Royal College of Physicians of Edinburgh. He was the 2005 recipient of the Rawls-Palmer Award and in 2008 received the honorary degree of doctor of laws, *honoris causa*, from the University of Dundee. Dr. Wood has served on a number of editorial boards, including that of the *New England Journal of Medicine*, and was the drug therapy editor of the *New England Journal of Medicine* from 1985 to 2004. His research has resulted in more than 300 articles, reviews, and editorials. He served on the U.S. Food and Drug Administration's Cardiovascular and Renal Drug Advisory Committee and the Non-Prescription Drug Advisory Committee, which he also chaired. He is currently the Chair of the Burroughs Welcome Fund Regulatory Science Award committee and serves on the board of the Critical Path Institute.

David W. Beier, JD, is managing director of Bay City Capital, a life sciences and drug development investment firm, which he has been with since 2013. He is a globally recognized leader in health care policy, pricing, intellectual property, government affairs, regulatory affairs, health care economics, and product commercialization. In addition, having spent two decades as part of the senior management teams for Amgen and Genentech, the two largest biotechnology companies in the world, he contributes invaluable perspective regarding strategy for entrepreneurial biotechs, the needs of potential acquirers, and the global health care industry in general. Mr. Beier served in the White House as the chief domestic policy advisor to Vice President Al Gore during the Clinton administration. He served as an appointee of President Clinton on his Advisory Committee for Trade Policy and Negotiations, on the Institute of Medicine (now Health and Medicine Division) panel on the Future of Health and Human Services, and as an advisor to the President's Council of Advisors on Science and Technology. Mr. Beier was also formerly a partner in the international law firm Hogan and Hartson and counsel to the U.S. House of Representatives Committee on the Judiciary. He has testified before Congress and the Federal Trade Commission; has written numerous law review articles and technical legal works; is regularly invited to author expert op-eds on health care; and has contributed to books on topics ranging from intellectual property to trade, privacy, and justice issues. He currently serves on the California State Government Organization and the Economy Commission, is a fellow of the Center for Global Enterprise, and teaches as an adjunct lecturer at the Haas School of Business at the University of California, Berkeley.

Thomas J. Bollyky, JD, is director of the global health program and senior fellow for global health, economics, and development at the Council on Foreign Relations (CFR). He is also an adjunct professor of law at Georgetown University. Mr. Bollyky is the author of *Plagues and the Paradox of Progress: Why the World Is Getting Healthier in Worrisome Ways* (MIT Press, 2018). He has written extensively on trade, health policy, and food and drug regulation, including on international regulatory cooperation and drug pricing. His expertise is in trade, health policy, and food and drug regulation. Prior to coming to CFR, Mr. Bollyky was a fellow at the Center for Global Development and a director at the Office of the U.S. Trade Representative (USTR), where he led the negotiations on medical technology regulation in the U.S.-Republic of Korea Free Trade Agreement and represented USTR in the negotiations with China on the safety of food and drug imports. He was a Fulbright scholar to South Africa, where he worked as a staff attorney at the AIDS Law Project, and an attorney at Debevoise & Plimpton LLP, where he represented clients before the International Court of Justice and the U.S. Supreme Court. Mr. Bollyky is a former law clerk to Chief Judge Edward R. Korman and was a health policy analyst at the U.S. Department of Health and Human Services. He has served in a variety of capacities at the National Academies, including as co-chair of its workshop on international regulatory harmonization and as a member of committees on strengthening food and drug regulation in developing countries and on the role of science, technology, and innovation in the future of the U.S. Agency for International Development. He has been a consultant to the Bill & Melinda Gates Foundation and a temporary legal advisor to the World Health Organization. In 2013, the World Economic Forum named Mr. Bollyky one of its global leaders under 40.

Katherine C. Bond, ScD, is vice president, international public policy and regulatory affairs, for the U.S. Pharmacopeia (USP). She develops and executes USP's global policy, advocacy, and regulatory affairs agenda in alignment with strategic organizational objectives and in support of medicines quality globally. Her expertise is in regulatory policy, systems strengthening, and cooperation, including medicines quality. Dr. Bond brings more than 25 years of demonstrated public health leadership experience—in the field and in management—having held positions at the U.S. Food and Drug Administration's Office of International Programs as associate director of technical cooperation and capacity building and director of the Office of Strategy, Partnerships, and Analytics. Prior to public service, Dr. Bond focused her energies on priority public health issues such as pandemics, infectious diseases, and health systems impacting Southeast Asia and Africa. She worked as associate director of The Rockefeller Foundation's Asia Regional Office and Africa Regional Office, and deputy director of the Mekong Regional Office of the Program for Appropriate Technology in Health. Dr. Bond has also held many consultancies and academic appointments—as both lecturer and researcher—at universities in the United States and abroad. She additionally appears as lead or contributing author on a variety of peer-reviewed research papers and technical documents in the areas of regulatory systems strengthening, global health security, health systems, and intervention strategies for specific at-risk populations.

Martha A. Brumfield, PhD, MS, is the former president and chief executive officer of Critical Path Institute, an Arizona-based nonprofit. In this role, Dr. Brumfield leads the institute in its mission to catalyze the development of new tools to advance medicine innovation and regulatory science, which is accomplished by leading teams that share data, knowledge, and expertise, resulting in sound, consensus-based science. Dr. Brumfield assumed the role of chief executive officer after most recently serving as the Critical Path Institute's director of international and regulatory programs. She also has her own consulting practice (Martha A. Brumfield LLC), focusing on concordance in global regulatory initiatives and regulatory science qualification programs. Other areas of focus in her practice include excellence in clinical trial conduct and pharmacovigilance, facilitation of scientific consortia, and programs supporting patient access to medicines. She is past chair of the board of directors for the Regulatory Affairs Professional Society and facilitated the Global Curriculum Coordinating Committee with the U.S. Food and Drug Administration's (FDA's) Office of International Policy, which developed a training curriculum framework for regulators in developing countries. She has worked with nonprofits such as GlobalMD to deliver educational workshops on regulatory and clinical trial topics in Asia. She has served on and contributed to Institute of Medicine consensus committees commissioned by FDA, focusing on global regulatory systems and on falsified and substandard drugs. She also serves on the steering committee of the Multi-Regional Clinical Trials Center of Brigham and Women's Hospital and Harvard. She is on the board of directors of the Institute for Advanced Clinical Trials for Children in Rockville, Maryland, and of Parkinson's Wellness Recovery in Tucson, Arizona. Dr. Brumfield brings 20 years of experience from Pfizer Inc., most recently as senior vice president of worldwide regulatory affairs and quality assurance. There, she led a global team that supported lifecycle pharmaceutical research, development, and commercialization through the creation and implementation of regulatory strategies and quality assurance oversight. Dr. Brumfield also played a key role in managing the broader company relationships with global regulators, trade associations, academics, and others on regulatory policy issues.

David Cockburn, BSc (Hons.), is the recently retired head of manufacturing and quality compliance with the European Medicines Agency (EMA). A pharmacy graduate, Mr. Cockburn has grounding in the pharmaceutical industry augmented by roles in the authorities at the national and European Union (EU) levels. Industry exposure included regulatory affairs at GD Searle and in production at Glaxo Operations, both in the United Kingdom (UK). Mr. Cockburn joined the UK Medicines & Healthcare products Regulatory Agency as a principal medicines inspector and spent 14 years there before moving to EMA for 15 years and becoming head of manufacturing and quality compliance. He worked part-time for the past 3 years of his career at EMA and during that time acted as the EU's technical lead in the process toward establishing the EU-US mutual recognition agreement on good manufacturing practice (GMP) inspections. Since retiring from EMA, Mr. Cockburn has formed associations with a number of organizations promoting training and education in GMP and medicines quality. Currently, these organizations comprise Pharma Consult Global and Euromed Communications as well as the European Qualified Persons

Association and University College London Innovation & Enterprise, which are nonprofit organizations.

Elizabeth Golberg, MA, recently completed a senior fellowship at the Mossavar-Rahmani Center for Business and Government at the Harvard Kennedy School. She retired in 2017 as director of better regulation at the European Commission and served as a member of the Organisation for Economic Co-operation and Development Regulatory Policy Committee in that capacity. Prior to that, she managed units in the European Commission's Secretariat General responsible for external relations G7/G20 and the president's briefings. In the early 2000s, she headed up a unit in the Environment Directorate General responsible for strategic planning and coordination. She held various advisory posts in the European Commission and was coordinator of the European Union's technical assistance program in the Czech Republic and Slovakia in the 1990s. She joined the European Commission in 1993, having served in the Canadian Foreign Service from 1980. Her areas of expertise are regulatory policy development and oversight, international regulatory cooperation, external relations, assistance in program coordination and management, and international trade.

Lawrence O. Gostin, JD, LLD, is university professor, Georgetown University's highest academic rank, conferred by the university president. Professor Gostin directs the O'Neill Institute for National and Global Health Law and is the founding O'Neill chair in global health law. He is professor of medicine at Georgetown University and professor of public health at Johns Hopkins University. Professor Gostin is the director of the World Health Organization (WHO) Collaborating Center on National and Global Health Law. He has also been appointed to high-level positions at WHO, such as the International Health Regulations Roster of Experts and the Expert Advisory Panel on Mental Health. He co-chairs the Lancet Commission on Global Health Law and is the legal and global health correspondent for the *Journal of the American Medical Association*. He is founding editor-in-chief of *Laws* (an international open-access law journal). He also holds multiple international academic professorial appointments, including at Oxford University, the University of Witwatersrand (South Africa), and Melbourne University. In 2016, President Obama appointed Professor Gostin to the National Cancer Advisory Board, on which he currently serves. He has expertise in such areas as health law and ethics, global health and global governance, AIDS law and ethics, human rights, privacy, and consent. In his previous positions, he served as associate dean for research at Georgetown Law; on the WHO director-general's Advisory Committee on Reforming the World Health Organization; and on numerous WHO expert advisory committees, including committees on the Pandemic Influenza Preparedness

Framework, smallpox, genomic sequencing data, and human rights. He served on the WHO/Global Fund Blue Ribbon Expert Panel: The Equitable Access Initiative, helping to develop a global health equity framework. He also served on the drafting team for the G7 Summit in Tokyo in 2016, focusing on global health security and universal health coverage. He was formerly the editor-in-chief of the *Journal of Law, Medicine & Ethics*. Professor Gostin served on the governing board of directors of the Consortium of Universities for Global Health. He is a member of the National Academy of Medicine.

Gavin Huntley-Fenner, PhD, is a human factors and safety consultant at Huntley-Fenner Advisors. His areas of expertise are risk management and communication. He has a unique problem-solving skillset and communication style developed over 20 years as a researcher, author, educator, and business consultant. He regularly provides consumer product hazard analyses and has served as an expert witness for matters relating to risk perception, instruction manuals, warnings, labeling, safety and human development, human reaction time, and decision making. Dr. Huntley-Fenner has been invited to speak at national and international scientific and non-scientific gatherings on topics ranging from basic and applied research, to forensic consulting, to education. He is a former member of the U.S. Food and Drug Administration's Risk Communication Advisory Committee.

Barbara Koremenos, PhD, MPP, is professor of political science at the University of Michigan. She received a National Science Foundation CAREER Award for her research—the first such winner to study international relations and law. She has given seminars in Canada, Denmark, France, Germany, Greece, Italy, Japan, Latvia, South Korea, Spain, Sweden, Switzerland, and the United States. Her award-winning book *The Continent of International Law: Explaining Agreement Design* (Cambridge University Press, 2016) focuses on how international law can be structured to make international cooperation most successful. She received her PhD from the University of Chicago.

Murray Lumpkin, MD, is deputy director, global health/integrated development, and lead for Global Regulatory Systems Initiatives at the Bill & Melinda Gates Foundation. The Global Regulatory Systems Initiatives are focused on working with partners such as the World Health Organization (WHO) (Geneva), the Pan American Health Organization, the WHO Regional Office for Africa, regulatory regionalization initiatives, and national regulatory agencies in all parts of the world to make more efficient and effective (without sacrificing product quality, efficacy, or safety) the regulatory processes through which health care products must pass to be developed, be eligible for procurement, and be legally marketed in low- and middle-income countries on which the Foundation focuses. Before joining the Bill & Melinda Gates Foundation, Dr. Lumpkin was director, Division of Anti-infective Drug Products (Center for Drug Evaluation and Research [CDER], U.S. Food and Drug Administration [FDA]); deputy center director for review management (CDER); and deputy commissioner for international programs at FDA. He served at FDA from 1989 to 2014.

Lembit Rägo, MD, PhD, is the secretary-general of the Council for International Organizations of Medical Sciences. He is also a current member of the World Health Organization (WHO) expert panel for the WHO Expert Committee on Pharmaceutical Specifications, which develops international drug quality assurance standards and guidelines. His research interests include international drug regulation, pharmaceutical policy, and regulatory cooperation. While previously at WHO, he worked on activities related to international nonproprietary names, quality assurance, pharmacovigilance, regulatory support, fighting falsified medicines, and prequalification of medicines. His previous positions include professor of clinical pharmacology at Tartu University; founder and first director general of the Estonian Drug Regulatory Authority, State Agency of Medicines; coordinator of the Quality Assurance and Safety: Medicines team at WHO; and head of WHO's Regulation of Medicines and Other Health Technologies unit.